The Pocket

FIRST-AID

FIELD GUIDE

Treatment and Prevention of Outdoor Emergencies

by George E. Dvorchak, Jr., MD

Skyhorse Publishing

Skyhorse Publishing books may be purchased in bulk at special discounts for sales promotion, corporate gifts, fund-raising, or educational purposes. Special editions can also be created to specifications. For details, contact the Special Sales Department, Skyhorse Publishing, 307 West 36th Street, 11th Floor, New York, NY 10018 or info@skyhorsepublishing.com.

Skyhorse® and Skyhorse Publishing® are registered trademarks of Skyhorse Publishing, Inc.®, a Delaware corporation.

Visit our website at www.skyhorsepublishing.com.

11

Library of Congress Cataloging-in-Publication Data

Dvorchak, George E.
 The pocket first aid field guide : treatment and prevention of outdoor emergencies / by George E. Dvorchak, Jr., M.D.
     p. cm.
   Includes bibliographical references and index.
   ISBN 978-1-61608-115-7 (pbk. : alk. paper)
 1. Outdoor medical emergencies--Handbooks, manuals, etc. 2. First aid in illness and injury--Handbooks, manuals, etc. I. Title.
   RC88.9.O95D86 2010
   616.02'52--dc22

                                                    2010010323

Printed in China

Photography Credits:
Photos: George Dvorchak
iStockphoto; *54, 76*
Scott Schupe: *80*

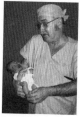

George E. Dvorchak Sr., MD

This book is dedicated to all physicians, nurses, medics, paramedics, EMTs and first-aid instructors. These individuals understand what it means to be first on the scene to render medical assistance. They know how to stabilize an injured person so he or she will survive to get to a medical facility. At the emergency room, skilled professionals use high-tech equipment and give it their all so someone who has been critically injured will survive.

One of these persons, a small town general practitioner, was my father, George E. Dvorchak, Sr. When accidents happened, be it in a local coal mine, at home or in the woods, Dad always did what he could with what he had available. Our rural area did not have emergency services beyond the hospital emergency room. The challenge was getting the victim from the field to the hospital, assisted by someone who knew basic first aid.

In those days, Dad did everything, from pulling teeth and making house calls to, at times, dealing with the medical needs of domestic animals. He even helped deliver me! If I got hurt, he would stop the bleeding and suture me. Dad was even on the teams that removed my tonsils and appendix.

I admired Dad for what he did and especially for being a good father, who also took the time to take me hunting and fishing and instilled in me confidence that helped me to survive.

CONTENTS

INTRODUCTION

If you get injured at home, knowing that help is a 911 phone call away is reassuring and certainly lifesaving. Accidents can happen anywhere, however, and especially in a wilderness setting, a minor injury can quickly become a major threat. When thrust into such a situation, the game plan for emergency help has suddenly changed and you are entirely on your own. Now what you must accomplish needs to be intelligently carried through if you or another injured person is to survive.

Because there are no books, videos or articles that can instantly make a physician out of anyone, I have written this book to serve as a reference to basic injuries with an emphasis on preventive medicine. Once you read this book, you will hopefully have a better idea of what precautions to take to minimize getting into a bad situation, especially in a wilderness environment where there isn't a medical facility available. If something should happen to you or a companion in such a locality, then through basic first-aid knowledge, you can make a difference by administering good, informed care. These first-aid tips should give you some direction in stabilizing various situations until trained medical personnel can be summoned to intervene and take that care to the next level.

As someone who has spent a lot of time in remote areas, I would also urge anyone contemplating an excursion into a territory where medical care is limited, or nonexistent, to seek advice from their family physician on medications, health precautions, vaccines or whatever medical advice "your" physician recommends to keep you healthy. After all, a good family physician will know his patient best and can therefore offer the best advice.

Also remember that if you are a hunter, or enjoy guided wilderness expeditions, you are well aware that it takes a good bit of money to go on a big game hunt or photo safari. By the time enough funds are available, you are usually older, and possibly, out of shape. Therefore, when you are selecting an outfitter or guide, seek one who is a good hunter and outdoorsman and is certified in CPR and first aid.

When booking, ask about emergency care options and their availability in his camp. Also, look for a wise outfitter who realizes that if a client is not 21 and tough as nails, he must adjust the hunting techniques or travel mode so as not to push that first time big game hunter or wilderness adventurer over the edge. When many of us look into the mirror, it becomes obvious that we may not be that kid we all once were, and adjustments in tactics are vital to avoid injury and stay healthy.

The world of the outdoors is beautiful and basically safe unless a major mistake is made. This usually happens when warning signs of impending danger are ignored. I am not talking about lurking grizzly bears or a looming avalanche, but of the warning signs in your body that may indicate that it is time to get a check-up. It is up to you to be educated to the point of being able to think ahead and take the necessary precautions that will help you to avoid injury or illness. If you think about the possible "what ifs," ahead of time, and something does happen, you will know what to do. Remember, your health and safety is up to you!

Having a basic knowledge of first aid can be helpful. It is the medical backup for prevention. If you can avoid an injury or accident, so much the better. If things go wrong a knowledge of basic first aid can be lifesaving. Remember, however, that doing something that could put an injured person at greater risk could be worse than doing nothing. A saying in medicine is to "do no harm!"

Over the years, I have observed that when an individual is faced with a tragedy and doesn't panic, you would be surprised what can be accomplished with basic knowledge and a cool head. To get to where you have this competence reguires a combination of basic knowledge and common sense.

This is why thinking through possible situations, carrying basic emergency gear and the knowledge of how to use it, gives you the tools you need to help yourself and others. With knowledge you can safely enjoy hunting, hiking or whatever you do in the great outdoors!

Neither the author nor the publisher can accept any responsibility for any loss, injury or damage caused as a result of the use or misuse of any practices or techniques described in this book, nor for any prosecutions or proceedings brought or instigated against any person that may result from using these practices or techniques.

THE AUTHOR

George E. Dvorchak, Jr., MA, MD is a recognized outdoor writer with articles on firearms, hunting, survival and outdoor medicine. Over the past 20 years, his health-related articles have been featured in national magazines such as *S.W.A.T.*, *American Survival Guide*, *Self Reliance Journal* and *Modern Survival*.

He is a contributing editor to *The Varmint Hunter* and *Modern Survival* magazines and has published articles in *Gun World*, *Guns*, *American Handgunner*, *Guns & Ammo*, *Safari*, *Shooter's Bible* and *Handguns*. He contributs to *Starzal* magazine in Poland and *Magnum* magazine in Brazil. George Dvorchak holds a bachelor's degree in education, a master's in human anatomy and an MD.

CONSULTANTS

Matthew J. Dvorchak, MD has provided direction concerning basic outdoors medical concerns and first aid from the standpoint of a physician and former emergency medical technician (EMT). He is active in his hometown fire company in Hastings, Pennsylvania, and is a board certified family practitioner, chairman of medicine at Miners Medical Center and medical director at HAIDA Manor in Hastings, Pennsylvania. His degrees include a bachelor's degree in biology and an MD.

Bernard H. DiGiacobbe, MD is chief of radiology at Tyrone Hospital in Pennsylvania and has provided insight into what certain injuries "look like" from the radiologist's point of view. He is also an authority on shotguns, double guns and drillings and is a contributing editor for *Shotgun Sports* magazine. As a small game hunter, he is also well aware of the potential for certain injuries when hunting or pursuing outdoor activities. He holds a bachelor's degree in biology and an MD.

Dennis P. Marcelli, D.D.S. provided practical information about dental problems. As an accomplished hunter and fisherman, he has spent a lot of time in camps. He is a family and cosmetic dentist with a bachelor's degree in biochemistry and a D.D.S. and resides in Jeannette, Pennsylvania.

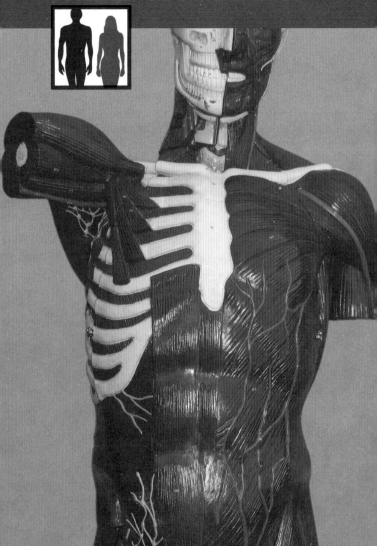

To better visualize underlying anatomy, the torso is divided into four quadrants. To better visualize this, imagine crossed lines that divide the torso into four parts. On the torso's right, the side with the arm pointing upwards, is the right upper quadrant (RUQ). The other side is the left upper quadrant (LUQ). Below the horizontal line passing through the umbilical, are the right lower (RLQ) and left lower (LLQ) quadrants. By knowing what organs are located under the skin in these areas, it becomes easier to pinpoint a suspected internal injury.

Some may open this book, look at the heading of the first chapter and ask themselves how a discussion of anatomy fits into a basic and practical approach to outdoor injuries and their prevention and treatment. Since anatomy is the branch of medical science that deals with the components and structure of the body, this discipline is the foundation for understanding both basic medicine and more about our own bodies and health. This knowledge becomes practical when there is visible trauma at a specific area on the "outside" of the body. At this point it is critical to understand what unseen structures lie beneath the concealing layers of hair, skin, fatty tissue and muscles. It is through an understanding of human anatomy that, when the body is traumatized and you can only see that one protective layer from the outside, that you can "see through" to the injury beneath. Understanding anatomy can help the observer make intelligent decisions as to how to approach the injury and deal with the situation.

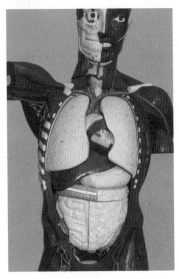

Now with the breast plate or skin and muscle removed, you can see what organs are located under the four quadrants.

Throughout this chapter, when I refer to man, it will be used to generally mean all the muscles, organs and other structures that function in unison to make up the entire individual. When all organs and systems function correctly, man will then be in the best of health possible for that individual's age and genetic make up, minus the disease states or disorders we acquire at times and simply have to live with.

Although not included in the discipline of pure anatomy, the topic of mental health is also important and can be related to physical disease and injury. Although it will not be discussed here, it will be slightly touched upon later in the chapter discussing stress. For now, this first chapter will concentrate on the physical aspects of the individual. Just remember that by knowing a little about how things work and where something is located underneath our outer protective layer, the skin, we will be in a better position if called upon to evaluate an injury to a human body.

Also, please bear with me in this first chapter since a fair amount of the information contained here goes beyond first aid. I firmly believe that this information is important, since by understanding more about the human body, you will find it easier to realize how the many smaller parts are related to others. With an understanding of these basic concepts, the how and why questions pertaining to our body, one's wellbeing and ultimately life itelf, are better appreciated.

THE HUMAN BODY

Most of us are usually born with two arms, two legs, a head, chest and abdominal area. Yet, it's critical for our health for all of the unseen organs to function as a team within our head and torso. Once you have covered this chapter and studied the photos of a torso and its divisions, you should then have a better idea of where organs are located and a better idea of what may be causing a particular pain or what organs could have been injured in an accident.

A severe injury to the limbs or other similar body parts is relatively easy to recognize. The revealed cross section of a severed or seriously severed foot or hand reveals fat, blood vessels, nerves, muscle and bone. These make up about half of our body's mass and the same holds true for both legs and arms. If a limb were severed, simply stopping or even slowing the bleeding and getting to a medical facility as quickly as possible would be your primary concern. With any injury where a lot of blood is lost, skilled medical intervention is the only prevention for shock, a condition that leads to organ failure and eventual death. If bleeding from a severed mangled arm or leg cannot be stopped, this is one of the few situations when a tourniquet should be applied. If an arm or leg is severed, as can be the case with a wound from a large caliber bullet, you need to prevent further loss of blood or that individual will go into shock and die. Generally speaking, if some part is severed from the body, do not leave that part behind, since with modern micro surgery techniques, severed limbs can often be reattached.

Another type of wound comes from a blow to the body or from being stabbed with something sharp. An injury from blunt trauma or a puncture wound becomes extremely critical when the organs of the human torso have been violated. Here, in order to establish what has been injured, with perhaps the exception of an injury to the heart and lungs' which can generally be easily determined, it is important to be able to look at a victim's torso and visualize what other organs may be situated under a specific wound.

To be able to refer medically and correctly to a particular part of the abdominal area, the abdominal region has been subdivided by anatomists into quadrants. To set the boundaries for this division, an imaginary line is drawn perpendicularly from the tip of the sternum (breastbone), called the xiphoid process, downward through the umbilicus (navel) to the pubic bone. To complete this division, another horizontal line, again crossing through the umbilicus, completes the sectioning. With these imaginary lines, the body has been mapped out for descriptive and location purposes. This gives us a better idea of what is in a specific area of the torso and therefore what was possibly injured.

There is nothing magical or particularly mysterious about this and how medical personnel use this information. To begin, since bits and pieces of knowledge make up small parts of the whole puzzle, a physician evaluates the type of pain, then introduces other factors, and, by correlating that knowledge with what he knows is located in a particular quadrant, gains a better idea of the causes of a particular pain or surface trauma. This seems simple but it is not, since the factor of REFERRED PAIN must be considered. Referred pain means that a painful sensation in one quadrant may have its source in another. This is where medical knowledge comes into play, since all of the signs and symptoms of disease or injury from an accident have to be logically sorted out along with any test data.

One last point to remember before beginning a discussion of the major organs concerns orientation. Always remember that when viewing a patient's torso, or an x-ray of the torso, right means the patient's right and left means his left, not yours. In other words, when viewing an x-ray film or looking at a patient, when you point to something on your left and the film's right, that is the patient's right side.

With the basic principles to understanding surface anatomy covered, I will now discuss the unseen major organs and their chief functions. Here is where basic physiology is helpful.

The Chest

Thoracic Cage – The upper part of the chest is covered and protected by 12 pairs of ribs. Ribs 1 to 7, known as true ribs, become progressively longer while the false ribs, beginning with rib number 8, become progressively smaller.

Their primary function is concerned with the protection and support of the underlying structures along with involvement in respiration. When you break or bruise a rib, as can be common in a fall or automobile accident, there will usually be severe pain at that site. Anyone who has broken a rib will know that simply taking a breath can be painful. In fact, if you fall out of a tree stand and experience pain when breathing, it is a good indication that a rib has probably been fractured. Despite the pain of a broken rib, the ribs' role in breathing is such that medical professionals recommended that, for a period of six weeks after the injury, you need to cough and take deep breaths once every hour to help prevent pneumonia.

A broken rib becomes particularly dangerous and

of immediate concern when a blow was so severe that the rib was broken and displaced. If this happens, you must consider what may have been severed or punctured in the underlying area. If there has been an injury or puncture of the lungs, the victim will usually cough up bright red blood that can also be frothy in appearance. Any deer hunter should recognize this sign since when trailing shot game, frothy blood is an indication of a lung shot.

Lungs – The lungs are the main organs of the respiratory system. Their task is to remove carbon dioxide from the blood while adding oxygen from the outside air. The lungs are normally soft and spongy. Within the thoracic cage, the lungs are divided into two halves, referred to as the right and left lobes. The right lobe is further divided into three lobes while the left is made up of two. The heart is located between the two major lobes and is partially protected in the front by the sternum and ribs.

Each lung is covered by a thin double membrane called the visceral pleura. Between this lining is fluid that provides lubrication to insure uniform and smooth expansion and contraction of the tissue during breathing. When this "lubricating area" becomes inflamed, a situation that can be caused by various conditions such as pneumonia or tuberculosis, it causes difficulty in breathing. This condition is called Pleurisy (an inflammation of the pleura). This is caused by excessive fluid accumulating in the pleura, compressing the lungs. (This is why a condition such as pneumonia is considered an emergency since it is difficult for a person to take a breath.) This condition is medically referred to as pleural effusion.

Another condition involving the lungs is called *Pneumothorax*. It comes about when the pleural cavity is compromised when air or gas enters it from the lungs or from outside the body. This can be caused by anything from a broken rib penetrating the lung (as in a fall from a tree stand) to a puncture wound caused by a knife or arrow. In some cases the cause of this condition can be difficult to determine since it can come about for no easily apparent reason.

Pneumonia is a common lung disorder that must be considered. It is an inflammation of the lungs that can have several causes. If you contract pneumonia in the wilderness, you may be in serious trouble, especially if you are alone, wet, cold and run down from exhaustion. Pneumonia is dangerous since this inflammation of the lungs can lead to death unless correctly diagnosed and treated with antibiotics (if the cause is bacterial). If you are concerned that you may have pneumonia, don't go out — rest and watch for signs that indicate that what you have is not simply a cold but something more serious. The warning signs and symptoms of pneumonia may be fever, chills and a cough that may produce greenish-yellow sputum. In the worse case one may even cough up blood. At the first signs or symptoms of pneumonia, immediately see your medical doctor for treatment. If you are in the wilderness, get to the closest emergency room as soon as possible.

Once you know where the lungs are located and understand their function, you have an understanding of what disorders can occur and will be better able to evaluate potential problems. Remember, the function of the lungs is to supply the cells of the body, through the blood, with oxygen while removing waste products such as carbon dioxide. The mechanism for this begins when air enters the body through the nose and mouth and filters down the trachea to the main bronchi. This process continues into the bronchioles and then into the small alveoli where the exchange of oxygen and carbon dioxide in the blood takes place.

You should be aware that if someone is not breathing, one of the tubes (trachea or bronchi), from the mouth to the lungs might be blocked as a result of a crushing injury or may be obstructed by something such as a bolus of food clogging the passage. It should be remembered that in CPR, one of the first steps is always to clear the mouth and tilt the head back before starting this life saving procedure. The lungs are necessary for life and any injury to them, or any potential infection is nothing to take lightly. In fact, seeking immediate medical intervention for a lung infection can prevent serious complications or, if there is an injury, it could be lifesaving.

Heart – The next vital organ located within the thoracic cage is the heart, our body's pump. This muscular pump is located under the sternum with its lower portion, medically referred to as the apex, located nearly under the left nipple. It takes this pump roughly a minute to completely circulate the body's 10 to 12 pints for a man or 8 to 9 pints of blood for a woman. To put this in perspective, when you donate blood, usually a pint is removed without resulting in problems since within a few hours, what was lost will be replaced. This replenishment is why you are given liquids to drink after donating blood.

Also do not overlook the pulse rate. This usually corresponds to the individual's heart rate and is important in giving clues to a person's state of health. Normal adult values range from 60 to 80 beats a minute with up to 120 to 140 being normal for a newborn.

Blood loss must be dealt with immediatly. It is obvious that even if the bleeding is stopped, lost fluids need to be replaced even if you are in a wilderness area away from medical care. After blood loss, you need to drink fluids.

The Four Areas of the Abdominal Area

For the purposes of reference we have divided the torso and its organs into four Quadrants:

RUQ
Right Upper Quadrant
- Majority of Liver
- Gallbladder
- Where Stomach Enters Duodenum
- Right Adrenal Gland
- Part of Right Kidney
- Colon's Hepatic Flexure
- Portions of Ascending & Transverse Colon

LUQ
Left Upper Quadrant
- Liver's Left Lobe
- Spleen
- Body of Pancreas
- Left Adrenal Gland
- Part of Left Kidney
- Colon's Splenic Flexure
- Portions of Transverse & Descending Colon

RLQ
Right Lower Quadrant
- Part of Right Kidney
- Appendix
- Cecum of Colon

LLQ
Left Lower Quadrant
- Part of Left Kidney

The area below the RLQ and LLQ contains
- Sigmoid Colon
- Part of Ascending Colon
- Part of Decending Colon
- Top Portion of Distended Urinary Bladder
- Right Ureter
- Left Ureter

In a Male: Right & Left Spermatic Cord
In a Female: Right & Left Ovary
- If Enlarged, the Uterus

Liver – Directly below the right lung is the Right Upper Quadrant (RUQ) which contains a large portion of a massive body organ, the liver. As a matter of fact, it is equal in mass to our skin. The role of this organ is to form products for blood coagulation, immunity and fat transportation (cholesterol). Besides this, it is also involved in the formation and excretion of bile used in digestion as well as the detoxification and excretion of toxic elements. (When you harvest an animal, it is always a good idea to examine the liver after field dressing since the liver can give you an indication of the animal's health.)

As with the heart, the liver is an organ critical to life. If it stops functioning from injury or disease, the result is death. The two diseases most commonly associated with it are hepatitis, which simply means that the liver is inflamed, and cirrhosis. Cirrhosis occurs when healthy cells are damaged, either as a result of poison, infection or some disease. In these cases, the healthy tissue is then replaced by scar tissue.

You should always be aware that hepatitis is an immediate threat while traveling in a third world country. There is no first-aid treatment for this condition and medical intervention is necessary. The first aid in this case is to be careful!

Gallbladder – Staying with RUQ, we find the gallbladder located under the liver. This pear-shaped sack measures between 6 to 10 cm long and can hold on the average of 45 ml of bile. Its fluid, when poured into the duodenum, aids in the digestion, emulsification and absorption of fats. A common disorder occurring within this organ is the formation of what are called gallstones. These "stones" may form as a result of the chemical composition of bile changing. When one of these stones becomes stuck in a duct, the resulting painful disorder is referred to as acute cholecystitis, meaning inflammation of the gallbladder.

Consideration of this organ should be of particular importance to anyone on high country hunts. In hunting camps, because of cold weather and a diet typically consisting of foods high in fat, persons predisposed to gallbladder problems may experience RUQ pain, nausea and vomiting. If you have such a concern, modify your diet and discuss this with your medical doctor since you may be having a problem with this organ. If it becomes severe, surgery may be indicated. Get this problem under control before you leave on a trip.

Spleen – This organ, the spleen, although non-vital, is located in the LUQ and is found between the fundus of the stomach and the diaphragm. Other organs adjacent to it are the left kidney, adrenal gland and lung.

The main function of the spleen is to remove worn out red blood cells from circulation, once their usefulness has ended after about 120 days. These cells, made in the bone marrow, are necessary to transport oxygen and nutrients. Even if a cell is not old, it is removed if it is damaged or defective.

An example of this is the disorder called sphe-rocytosis. This disorder is caused by many small, round red blood cells called spherocytes. Since these blood cells are abnormal, they are fragile and break up when passing through the spleen. Remember, although it is the spleen's function to remove such abnormal cells, these brittle cells easily break up in a process referred to as hemolysis. Since red blood cells (needed to carry hemoglobin to transport oxygen), are destroyed at a rate that exceeds the production of new cells in the bone marrow, the overall result is anemia. In this situation, the treatment for spherocytosis is to remove the spleen.

Be aware that if the spleen is ruptured, by a severe blow for example, a lot of blood will be lost. This internal bleeding can be critical! When this happens, you can now logically understand its connection with blood and why one bleeds a lot when the spleen is ruptured. Being in an automobile accident or kicked in that area by a horse is a sure way to get into trouble. Due to its position, in the case of an abdominal injury where ribs are broken on the left, the spleen is frequently ruptured as a result of crushing forces.

Stomach – The stomach, also located in the LUQ, is situated under the diaphragm. It is a sack-like hollow organ that expands as one fills up on food and drink. It is in the stomach where foods are broken down by gastric juices. Within the stomach, glands that secrete mucus provide the lining with protection from these juices.

We can get into trouble when the lining of the stomach is attacked by hydrochloric acid forming a crater called a Peptic Ulcer. This condition becomes particularly dangerous if you are not aware of its presence.

Take the activity of a wilderness hike or hunt for example. After 8 to 10 hours of walking or horseback riding, you will definitely be sore. Perhaps by evening, to be able to sleep, you take a medication to kill the pain. Here is where trouble can begin! With ulcers, one should not risk drinking alcohol or taking medications for pain that contain aspirin since these medications can accelerate damage to a peptic ulcer.

This is also where arthritic sufferers, due to their reliance on medications for pain and inflammation, must be careful with their medications at all times, especially when they are beyond easy access to medical facilities. With time and knowledge, individuals so affected learn to take such medication only with food so to add some protection to the stomach. If you suffer from muscular aches and pains, be careful what you take to alleviate them.

Small Intestine – The small intestine has an average length of 22 feet and is found in all four quadrants. The first part of the small intestine extends from the point where the stomach empties into it, called the duodenum (about 10 inches long), to where it empties into the colon or large intestine. This last section is roughly 12 feet long and is called the ileum. The center section, about 10 feet long, is referred to as the jejunum.

Colon – The large tube of the digestive system, the colon, will have a length of about 6 feet and is found in all parts of the abdominal quadrants. It begins, in the RLQ near the appendix and is called the cecum. From that point going upwards, the colon is referred to as the ascending colon.

In continuing upwards near the right lobe of the liver, it turns to the left crossing the abdomen from left to right and is referred to as the transverse colon. On the left side, beneath the lower margin of the spleen, the colon flexes downward and is now referred to as the descending colon. From here it enters the pelvis and, in that location, is called the sigmoid colon. Then, continuing downward to the tube's end, we have the rectum.

Common disorders affecting this system can be anything from cancer to ulcerative colitis and diverticular disease. A disorder that you should be aware of, one that frequently has a sudden onset, is acute appendicitis. When the appendix, a mystery organ with no apparent function, becomes inflamed and filled with puss, a victim can be in severe pain that may have started around the navel and eventually settles in the RLQ.

A person suffering from acute appendicitis may become nauseous, vomit and have an urge to pass gas or a stool. In a worse case scenario, the appendix ruptures. In this case, the severe pain usually subsides but the possibility of developing a serious disorder, called peritonitis, an inflammation of the lining of the abdominal cavity, may develop. If you suspect appendicitis, get the victim to medical assistance as soon as possible.

A common disorder of the *anorectal area* are hemorrhoids. These are dilated veins that can become swollen and can cause bleeding. If you suffer from hemorroids, or are concerned that you may have them, consult with your physician before a wilderness trip. He can suggest medications to have on hand to be used in an emergency.

Located in the RUQ is the head of the pancreas. The body of this gland is located posterior to the stomach in the LUQ. Its tail, or narrower portion, ends near the spleen. The pancreas serves exocrine and endocrine glandular functions which perform hormonal and digestive jobs.

Included among the endocrine functions are the Islets of Langerhans, which secrete the hormones insulin and glucagon. These regulate the levels of glucose in the blood. When one suffers from *Diabetes Mellitus,* these insulin producing cells are destroyed and insulin is no longer available as a source of energy. When the brain is cut off from nutrients, the result can be dangerous conditions such as a coma.

Once you are aware that you have diabetes, there is no reason why, with good medical care and a willingness to take an active role in that care, that you cannot lead an active and normal life. Unfortunately, some diabetics keep their disorder to themselves. While this may be personal information, it should not be a secret when on a wilderness excursion.

When a guide or others are aware that one of their number has this specific medical disorder, they can make accomodations and have an understanding of what symptoms to monitor and what actions to take if there is a diabetic emergency.

If you have a weight loss despite having a good appetite, suffer from increased urination and thirst, fatigue, impotence, blurred vision, wounds or sores that do not heal or other conditions that you or family members see as abnormal, get to your doctor for an evaluation. One of the possible causes could be a problem with your pancreas that might lead to diabetes mellitus. Check out such medical concerns before going on any outdoor trip since what may be shrugged off as simply not feeling good might be something that can be corrected if caught before serious consequences develop.

Kidneys – Next, there are two organs about 5 inches long that are located between the lower and upper quadrants, our right and left kidneys. The one on the right is under the liver while the one on the left is under the spleen. Because of the size of the liver on the right, the kidney under it is positioned a little lower than the one on the left.

The functions of these organs is to filter blood and excrete the waste products and excess fluid as urine. The kidneys are also important in controlling the balance between acid and base in the body's system along with regulating electrolytes (the substances that transmit electricity in our bodies).

When one or both of your kidneys are damaged by various infections, the disorder is referred to as pyelonephritis. Other causes of kidney disorders can be tumors, trauma as from an accident, kick, punch, fall or medical disorders as diabetes mellitus, hypertension or others.

Two glands, the adrenals, are located on top of the kidneys. These secrete certain important hormones directly into the blood circulation. Tumors, Cushing's or Addison's disease are disorders that are associated with the adrenals.

Urinary Bladder – This hollow organ is the reservoir for our urine and is connected to the kidneys by a tube called the ureter. When the bladder fills up (it contains around a pint of liquid), the urine is excreted through another tube called the urethra. The urethra is about 8 inches long in the male and about 2 inches in females. When this reservoir becomes infected, we have a condition known as cystitis. Due to the shorter tube in females, women have a greater tendency for bladder infections than men.

If a blunt trauma occurs to the pubic area, the bladder may rupture, especially if it is full at the time the blow occurs. If this medical emergency happens and the symptoms seem to include more than surface bruising, the results may be serious and potentially life threatening. It is best to get the victim to medical care as soon as possible.

2. PHYSICAL CONDITIONING

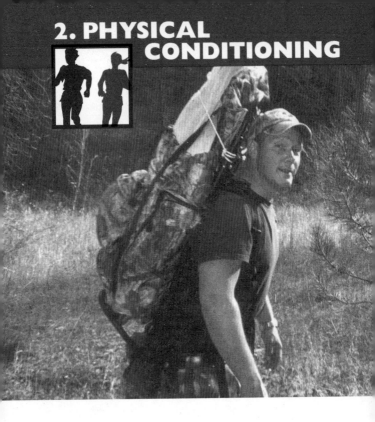

An intelligent approach to exercise is something that should concern all of us. If we are in good physical shape, we are less likely to "stress out" and get our bodies into difficult situations. The problem might be as simple as participating in a hike and discovering that even moderate exercise is exausting and you are unable to continue.

On the other hand, the situation might be dire.

The hunter at left, Augie Reich, is shown packing out the meat, cape and antlers from a 5 x 5 bull elk. In order to pack out the meat and his gear, Reich had to carry several loads on his back for about 3.5 miles. In total, it took him five round trips, a total of 35 miles. Fortunately Reich was prepared for this by prior physical conditioning through a well planned exercise routine.

The chest pains that you experience as a result of the exertion on your hike may be an indication that you have pushed an out-of-shape body into a heart attack. Remember, being prepared doesn't simply mean buying the right equipment. You also have to be physically ready to handle the exertions that you will encounter in the outdoors. Before starting any exercise program, however, it's a good idea to consult with your physician and get a check-up so you can start your exercise program without getting into trouble.

KEEPING FIT

Among America's older population, there are many individuals who, for a considerable period of their life, are only concerned with work and have little or no time for "play." Eventually they become established and successful, say in their 40s or 50s, and finally have some time and "extra" cash to devote to that diverted "play."

For many, play/exercise involves physical activities such as hiking, bike riding, jogging and, for those who hunt, possibly a first and only big game excursion into the back country where your two feet and possibly a horse are the only means to get around. Being an avid hunter and spending a lot of time "out there," I have witnessed many individuals who have gotten into trouble – even some where the outcome was death. For many, a strenuous vacation in wild country can be a satisfying and relaxing experience, but for those in poor shape, what should have been a rewarding experience might suddenly turn into a disaster.

In the wilderness, problems can arise, particularly in fall and winter months, since at that time of the year we are exposed to the one of the many risk factors for heart attack (myocardial infarction) – extreme cold. In the case of an individual who is a little overweight or who smokes, we can add exertion/excitement to that environmental extreme. With that they may find that the cards are beginning to stack-up against their survival.

Physical Exam

Before participating in any strenuous physical activity, to play it safe, check with your medical doctor and tell him that you want to begin an exercise program to get in shape. You do not want to begin what could be a good program only to learn that you have a hidden medical problem that turns what should have been beneficial into a situation that might kill you or put you in the hospital. At your physical, your physician will question you to compile a medical history and perform an examination (the physical). All of this medical information combined with lab data from tests will be interpreted to offer a good idea of what you can and cannot do safely. With this information you can safely begin a program with the least amount of risks to you.

Remember, getting "checked out" is simply a form of preventative medicine since many diseases and disorders become more prevalent as we age. As we get older, what may have been latent surfaces over time. Early detection and follow-up treatment and/or occupational modification can slow the progression of a disease or completely eliminate an unexpected risk. It is up to you! To give you some idea of what to expect, the following is an example of how such an exam will progress.

Skin, Hands & Nails – These are evaluated for color, temperature, texture, moisture, vascularity, deformities and the presence of lesions.

Head – A funduscopic exam of the eyes looks for microaneurysms, arteriolar changes or the presence of exudates (material formed by a discharge of fluid and cells from blood vessels onto the surface of the eye causing inflammation). This reveals hemorrhages from hypertension or diabetic retinopathy (damage to the retina from diabetes).

Ears – An otoscopic exam checks for hearing loss, otitis media (middle ear inflammation) or any sensory-neural disorder.

Nose – Check the nasal passages for polyps or lesions.

Neck – The neck is examined for masses along the lymph nodes. The thyroid is palpated (felt) for masses which could be nothing or something severe as a tumor. The carotid arteries in the neck are auscultated (listened to) with a stethoscope in an effort to pick-up sounds that could indicate a blockage in these important arteries.

Chest: Lungs & Heart – Check for obstructive lung disease that can present problems during high country (high altitude) trips. A chest x-ray will evaluate risk factors for smokers or persons working under "high risk" conditions. A pulmonary function test tells how the lungs are functioning.

A stethoscopic evaluation will look for problems with a valve or conducting system (regulates the beats of the heart). An EKG test records the electrical impulses of the heart muscle. Abnormal patterns can indicate coronary heart disease, coronary thrombosis (a blockage), pericarditis (inflammation of the membrane that surrounds the heart), myocarditis (heart inflammation) and arrhythmia (abnormal heart rhythms).

Abdomen – The abdomen will be checked for hernia, a protrusion of an organ (the intestine pushing through a week abdominal muscle). With strenuous activity it could strangulate.

You will also be evaluated for ulcers. A peptic ulcer occurs in the esophagus, stomach or small intestine or duodenum when the stomach's lining is broken down or eroded by excessive acid or infection. To avoid severe pain and complications from a perforation or bleed, avoid aspirin that can precipitate damage to a sensitive stomach and modify diet to avoid pain and complications while in the back country.

Rectum – A colon digital (finger length) exam looks for masses (tumors) and, on men, also checks the prostate. Check for occult (hidden) blood in the stool. Examine for hemorrhoids.

Musculoskelatal System – You will be examined for arthritis and disk disorder. A careful and proper diagnosis is critical to avoid emergencies. It is a good idea to evaluate any pains to rule out dangerous specific causes.

Review Your Medications

Discuss the medications you may be taking with your physician and then have sufficient amounts for your trip. Make a list of medications and carry it with you along with the phone number of your physician. It is also a good idea to let anyone who may be accompanying you know what medications you are taking.

At times, especially if you are staying at a lodge, alcohol will be available. Be aware that mixing alcohol with various medications, either prescription or over-the-counter, can be dangerous. For example, you might choose acetaminophen (Tylenol) after a long day in the field for sore muscles. The combination can cause liver damage. Also, cold preparations contain antihistamines and these have a sedative effect. It is simply a good idea not to take any medication with any drink containing alcohol.

Getting Into an Exercise Routine

Now that you have been evaluated by your physician as to the risks of beginning a program, here are some suggestions on how to slowly get back on track.

Setting Goals – Set up a program tied to your planned outdoor activity and design your exercise program according to what you wish to accomplish. This can include such factors as weight loss, improving endurance and/or strength, or a host of other reasons.

Establishing Goals – Being specific in establishing realistic short and long-term goals is important to keeping on track as long as you don't confuse the objectives and become discouraged. For example, if your "goal" is losing weight, this can be a slow and often frustrating process and can take time and considerable effort to accomplish.

To get started, you need a short term goal, say to drop 2 pounds a week. This is achievable with a sensible diet tied to exercise. Two pounds a week is realistic where that 60 pound figure seems so far away. Don't become discouraged from the start. Think small and take it from there with a realistic approach to achieving your goals.

Endurance – Cardiovascular conditioning

is what this is all about. According to the book, *Primary Care Secrets*, intensity, duration and frequency are the factors that should be incorporated into your exercise programs. It is stated that the "intensity of exercise (should be) in the range of 50-80 percent of maximal oxygen uptake which corresponds to 65-90 percent of the maximal heart rate. This is approximately equal to 220 minus the person's age."

To get your target heart rate, for a sedentary person age 60, take the 220 and subtract 60 (age) times .65, which equals 104 beats per minute, which is the targeted heart (pulse) rate. For duration (length of time to exercise) and frequency (how often), "15 to 45 minutes of exercise 3 to 5 times a week are generally recommended." Brisk walking is the ideal beginning exercise. Fast walking and biking are good starts. Later, it may be advisable to switch over to jogging. This is a good exercise but can put stress on your joints.

Stairs – At work, skip the elevator and take the stairs. When exercising outside, be careful during any activity in hot or cold weather since these conditions contribute to strain on anyone, particularly those not in shape, so be careful. Also, especially on a hot day, carry water and keep yourself hydrated. Getting dehydrated is another of those conditions that can hurt us and can happen before we are aware.

Swimming – Unlike jogging, swimming does not put strain on one's ankles and joints. Unfortunately, not everyone has access to swimming facilities.

Bicycling – I personally prefer this as an exercise, at least when there is no snow on the ground. It provides excellent benefits to the cardiovascular systems, and burns calories. It also increases both muscle tone and leg muscle strength and a ride through pleasant surroundings is quite relaxing and eliminates stress.

On the negative side, (one reason why a stationery bike at home may be better for some), road riding can be dangerous. Always wear a helmet and check out the air quality index for pollutants and pollen before you go. Check out your local park service for information on bike and walking trails. Due to the increased popularity of exercise, many areas of the country have specific trails for walking, jogging or biking. I prefer these since I do not want to be on a highway competing with motorized vehicles for space.

Weight and Strength Training – Weight training should be approached with caution to avoid injuries. Before starting weights, get checked out by a physician and only then begin an exercise routine. I recommend beginning with endurance exercises. Later, continue with these but add weights.

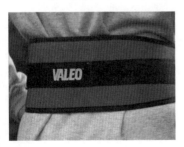

To avoid a rupture or back injury when participating in weight and strength training, wear a back brace.

Consider going to a gym with qualified trainers who can provide advice on starting a program. These men and women can develop a plan specific to your needs while minimizing the risk of injury. Play it safe and get all the help that is available since the right program will lessen the possibility of injuries. But remember, the key to success is *not quitting*. Stick with it but don't overdo it. Consider exercising daily but not the same muscle groups. By this I mean to do aerobic or endurance exercises such as fast walking or biking every other day and use weights on opposite days.

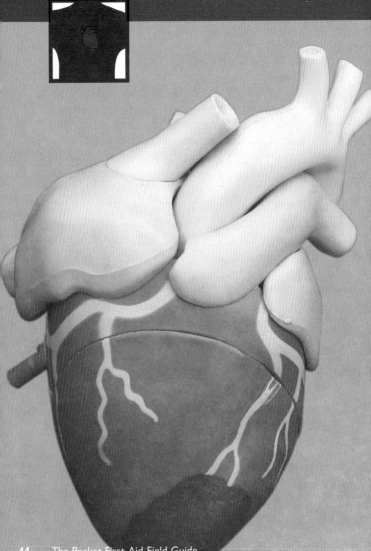

*The dark area on the bottom of this model of a
heart represents dead muscle. The tissue destruction
is from coronary arteries being blocked and therefore, oxygenated blood can not supply the muscle
with life sustaining blood. When the heart muscle is
damaged, pumping blood is no longer efficient.*

According to the book *Primary Care Secrets*, every
year almost a million individuals die from diseases
of the heart in the United States. This number is
drawn from the estimated 70 million individuals
who have risk factors for coronary heart disease,
high blood pressure and stroke.

When considering coronary heart disease
(CHD) – any damage to the heart caused by a
narrowing or blockage of the coronary arteries
– it is estimated that nearly 12 million Americans
are affected in one way or another. If you are one
of these high risk individuals, however, statistics
mean little and you know all to well that you have
a serious problem!

In knowing this, the health conscious individual
will begin to wonder if there is anything that can
be done to keep himself out of that high-risk population. To present this information, I believe that
the best approach is to list the risk factors and
their importance. If you fit in any of these groups,
be aware that you may have a problem and take
precautions to avoid the eventual causes of heart
disease. Remember, heart disease is not a death
sentence and with proper management, including

lifestyle changes, you can generally resume a normal life and participate in outdoor activities as well.

MAJOR RISK FACTORS FOR ATHEROSCLEROTIC CARDIOVASCULAR DISEASE

Fixed Risk Factors

Age – As we age, there are changes in our organs and their structure. With age, the heart muscle becomes less elastic and loses efficiency. The heart can also atrophy with age! With certain diseases, however, the heart can enlarge and not function properly.

Hypertension – Another change involves the blood vessels which become less elastic with age. It becomes harder for the heart to pump blood efficiently (circulate). With less elasticity in the arteries and blood vessels, blood pressure increases. An aging heart and vascular can be likened to a

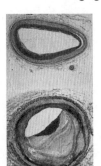

sump pump and outlet hose. During cold weather (age), the outside line can freeze almost completely (think of this as clogged arteries). When the sump pump turns on and tries

The coronary artery on the top is open and allows blood to move unobstructed. That partially blocked on the bottom, which restricted blood flow, is closing in on life. With the heart, a muscle, needing more oxygen during exercise, that vessel with a small opening can not deliver enough blood carrying oxygen with the result being chest pains and even a heart attack.

to pump water through a nearly clogged line, the pump now has to work a lot harder for a longer time. As a result, it heats up and finally fails. When the heart cannot circulate blood through plugged vessels, a similar outcome ensues. In the body, the condition of narrowed or constricted blood vessels is called *Arteriosclerosis*. When the coronary vessels narrow, less oxygen reaches the heart (a muscle requiring oxygen like any other) resulting in Angina (pain) or a heart attack.

Sex – Males are at a greater risk along with postmenopausal females.

Heredity – You are at risk if there is a family history of premature coronary heart disease.

Modifiable Risk Factors

These risk factors are largely under your control. In some cases, you cannot work hard and "cure" the problem or medical condition, but, through certain lifestyle changes, an individual may be able to keep the situation under control.

Smoking – The habitual use of tobacco can be both the easiest and one of the hardest heart-risk factors to control. If you really want to break the addiction, consultation with a good physician along with family support can help.

High Cholesterol & Triglycerides – This is a condition that a good and aggressive physician can help you to keep within or close to safe limits. Here, diet modification is critical along with the important element of adding fiber.

There are things you can do if your triglycerides are over 200 mg/dl. If you are overweight, try to lose sufficient weight to get close to the average ideal weight for your body type. Also, limit alcohol intake. If you are a diabetic, work at keeping your condition under control.

If your cholesterol numbers are high and diet does not seem to be helping, then your physician may elect to put you on a medication to help lower cholesterol, reduce the LDL ("bad" artery-clogging cholesterol) and increase HDL ("good" cholesterol). Don't expect immediate results but keep on the schedule outlined by your doctor and don't give up.

Diet, possible medications and getting away from a sedentary lifestyle, the easiest risk factor to modify, should fit into your "treatment" regime. Remember, sitting behind a desk puts few demands on your body's cardiovascular system.

Once cleared by your doctor, aerobic exercise phased in gradually to avoid injury, will begin to make you feel better. Your heart becomes more efficient through exercise, and effects on any rising cholesterol.

Obesity – Exercise also affects another potentially modifiable risk, obesity. An estimated 20-30 percent of the United States population is affected. Along with heredity, other factors such as hypothyroidism, tumors of the adrenal gland, pituitary or pancreas or emotional factors can cause obesity. Being overweight is an important factor contributing to heart disease due to its association with high cholesterol levels in the blood. Overweight individuals tend to have lower HDL ("good" cholesterol) levels.

Managing diet and avoiding obesity can contribute to avoiding Diabetes Mellitus, a disorder where the pancreas produces insufficient or no insulin and causes the level of glucose in the blood to increase. Obesity plays a significant role since it is a primary cause of unmasking latent diabetes. This condition is dangerous if it is allowed to get out of control it can be responsible for the lipid metabolism being out of order and can contribute to an accelerated degeneration of the body's small blood vessels.

Diet & Body Fat – How do we reduce body fat through diet? Basically, reduce fat, sodium, overall calorie intake and sugar in the diet. It is also a good idea to increase fiber. Eat at regular intervals, watch what you eat (especially fast foods), don't snack and add exercise. Remember you didn't become overweight over night and don't expect to take off 20 pounds in a week.

After loosing weight, the key is in keeping it off! Remember, contributing factors to obesity are diet, physical inactivity and in some cases, heredity. Even if you can't do anything about your ancestry, don't use the heredity factor as a crutch and do nothing!

Most risk factors can be modified with a little work. While these solutions are not directly considered first aid, they are measures that will help avoid heart problems.

4. BREATHING & CHOKING

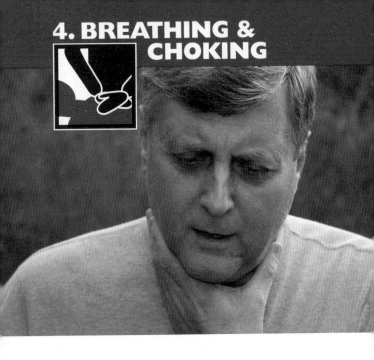

Breathing difficulties can be the result of a wide range of causes ranging from asthma and allergic reactions (anaphylactic shock) to injury and heart attack. Whatever the cause, dificulty breathing, except perhaps for feeling slightly winded from normal activity, is always a medical emergency. If you encounter a person who is not breathing you will need to take immediate action. A person can survive a considerable blood loss or severe dehydration, but without oxygen, the body and brain will die in a very short period of time. When the victim of an illness or accident is not breathing,

The posture of the person at left is a common sign that someone is choking. Their hand or hands may be at their throat with their thumb and fingers extended as shown. This is the universal sign of choking and indicates that this person needs help!

you will have to "breathe" for them and begin first aid in the form of rescue breathing.

RESCUE BREATHING

- Check to see if the person is breathing normally.
- Make sure that the person's airway is open. Tilt their head back by lifting the chin with one hand, while pressing down on the forehead with the other hand.
- Look for an obstruction. If one is present, try to remove it with your fingers.
- Place your ear next to the victim's mouth and nose and listen for any sounds of breathing, feel for air movement on your cheek and look to see if the chest is rising.
- If you don't perceive signs of normal breathing, you must breathe for the victim.
- Tilt the victim's head back, place your mouth over the victim's mouth and pinch the victim's nose closed. Breathe into their mouth slowly two times, making sure that their chest rises with each breath.
- Give 10 breaths and check the person's pulse. If there is no pulse, CPR may be needed.

CPR

WARNING: This is intended as a guideline for learning about CPR only! It is not intended to replace formal CPR training. Contact the American Heart Association or the Red Cross to find out about a CPR course. Never practice CPR on another person, without proper training.

Chest Compressions – If there are no signs of normal breathing, begin chest compressions.

- Place the heel of one hand on the middle of the victim's chest on the center of the sternum. Place the heel of your other hand on top of the first hand. Lock your elbows and place your shoulders directly above your hands.
- Press down on the chest with sufficient force to move the breastbone down about 2 inches.
- Compress the chest 30 times, at a rate of about 100 times per minute.
- After 30 compressions, stop, check the airway, and give 2 slow breaths.
- Reposition your hands in the same spot and perform another 30 chest compressions. Repeat the 30 compressions and 2 breaths for 4 cycles, or about 1 minute.
- After about 1 minute of CPR, stop and check to see if the person has started breathing normally. If not, continue CPR until help arrives. This technique is used on anyone older than 8 years.

CHOKING

Once the respiratory passage becomes blocked, most commonly by a bolus of food, one begins to choke. To stop choking and dislodge any obstruction in the breathing passage, you should learn how to perform the Heimlich maneuver.

Emergency First Aid for Choking
Heimlich Maneuver
- Stand behind the person and wrap your arms around their waist.
- Make a fist and position it just above the person's bellybutton.
- Grasp the fist with the other hand and with a quick upward thrust, push hard into that area of the abdomen.
- If nothing flies out their mouth and the victim is still choking, repeat the action. It may take more than one time to remove the obstruction.

Choking if You are by Yourself
If this happens, all is not lost since you can make a fist and thrust it into your abdomen yourself. Another option is, with your fist positioned over the abdomen, drape yourself over something hard such as a chair or log as you push up with your hand.

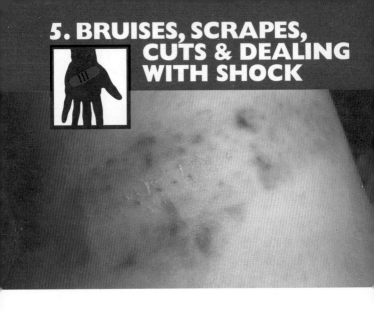

5. BRUISES, SCRAPES, CUTS & DEALING WITH SHOCK

When incisions and lacerations go beyond the outer layer of skin and into the deeper layers that contain blood vessels, severe bleeding can result. Major bleeding is always a life-threatening condition that requires immediate attention. Major blood loss can quickly lead to shock and death.

BLEEDING

Bleeding may be the result of a severed artery, vein or capillary.

- **Arterial Bleeding** – This type of bleeding spurts with each beat of the heart, is bright red in color and is severe and hard to control. Move immediatly to stop arterial bleeding.

- **Venus Bleeding** – characterized by a steady flow; the blood is a dark shade. This is easier to control than arterial bleeding.
- **Capillary Bleeding** – slow, oozing bleeding

Emergency First-Aid Treatment for Bleeding

- Have the injured person lie down and, if possible, position their head slightly lower than the torso and elevate the legs. This position increases the blood flow to the brain and reduces the risk of fainting and shock.
- If possible, elevate the site of the wound.
- If you can, remove any observable debris or dirt from the wound. Don't try to pull out any large or deeply embedded objects.

Direct Pressure

- Apply direct pressure to the wound using a sterile bandage or clean dry rag, towel or piece of clothing. If you have nothing else, you can use your hand.
- Keep up the pressure until the bleeding stops. Hold continuous pressure for at least 20 minutes.
- Maintain pressure by applying a tight bandage (or even a section of clean clothing) over the wound.
- After applying the bandage, check the pulse to make sure circulation is not interrupted. A slow pulse rate or bluish fingertips or toes are warning signs that a bandage may be blocking

circulation. Don't remove the gauze or bandage
even if the bleeding continues and seeps into
the material you are holding on the wound.
Add more material over the original dressing.

Pressure Points

If you can't stop the bleeding with direct pressure,
apply pressure to the artery that carries blood to
the area of the wound. These "pressure points"
are located on the:

- **Arm** – On the inside of the wrist (radial
  artery where the pulse is checked) and on
  the inside of the arm just above the elbow
  and under the armpit (brachial artery)
- **Leg** – Just behind the knee and in the crease
  in the groin (femoral artery)

Press the main artery in these areas against
the bone, keeping your fingers flat. At the same
time, keep up pressure on the wound location. Don't move the injured body part once
the bleeding has stopped. Leave the bandages
in place and get the injured person to professional medical help.

HYPOVOLEMIC SHOCK

The next topic I would like to mention, since
it is usually associated with a loss of blood, is
Hypovolemic Shock. Although there are other
types of shock, that caused by blood loss is the
most common resulting from the type of injury

most likely to occur in the outdoors. Due to severe blood loss, the circulatory system collapses and the victim may become comatose. This is serious since if it is not recognized and reversed, the result could be deadly. To identify shock, you need to know what to look for.

Symptoms of Shock
- Skin – pale in color with a cold and clammy feeling
- Pulse – located on the thumb side of the inner wrist, is weak and rapid
- Blood pressure – low
- Breathing – rapid and shallow
- Consciousness – The individual is confused, faint and weak or unconscious.

Emergency First-Aid Treatment for Shock
For this medical emergency, you must check breathing and stop any bleeding.
- Lie the victim down and, if possible, slightly elevate the feet while keeping movement to a minimum. In this position, blood flow to the head is maximized. Try to loosen any constricting clothing.
- If it is cold out, keep the person warm by covering him with a blanket. Also put something beneath the individual to prevent heat loss to the ground. If it is hot out, keep them out of the hot sun and rest on a blanket.

- Put the person on their side to prevent choking from aspiration of stomach contents. To
  prevent vomiting, avoid giving the victim anything to drink even if he states he is thirsty.
- Summon medical help as soon as possible.

WOUNDS

The tissue that covers our body (skin) has the
important function of protecting the internal
organs and tissues from the "outside" environment
and penetration by physical objects. This protective covering is our largest body organ and the
body's first line of defense against injury, dirt and
bacteria. With any injury, the outer layer of skin,
the epidermis, is either scraped away or opened
up which, while it may seem superficial, permits
bacteria and materials to enter the system. In a
more severe wound, the next layer downward, the
dermis, is penetrated. The dermis contains connective tissue, sweat glands, hair follicles, nerves,
lymph and blood vessels. Generally speaking, the
deeper the wound, the more serious the consequences it can have for the body.

Wound Management

The first concern with any wound is to control bleeding. On the first-aid level, this usually means through
the use of a pressure bandage. The next concern is to
prevent wound contamination which refers to cleaning the wound and applying a sterile bandage and

possibly an antibiotic ointment. Lastly, immobilization of the injured part along with rest and if severe, medical intervention, are the procedures to follow.

Closed Wounds to the Skin

This is the common bruise or contusion which is generally caused by a blunt object impacting the body. The result is that blood will begin to leak from the injured vessels under the skin which causes a surface area to change color to a black or blue shade. Since the skin has not been broken, there is less chance of infection. The immediate first-aid treatment is to apply ice, or a "cool pack" for about 10 minutes and then periodically throughout the day to reduce swelling and pain.

Even though the skin has not been broken, a bruise or contusion can be a serious problem depending on the amount of force that caused the injury and what organs are located under that area that might have been injured as well.

Here is where knowledge of surface anatomy is important when evaluating an injury. For example, if an internal organ in the abdominal area has been severely injured, bleeding may be taking place internally without external evidence. When riding or hunting with horses, an internal blunt force injury could be caused by a kick to the abdomen. A hiker might fall heavily on a projecting rock. In these and similar cases, an internal injury could result.

Be careful in such situations when you are hours

or even days from medical care. Internal bleeding can be fatal. Remember, not all injuries are obvious so look beyond the obvious and try to get a potential victim to medical assistance if possible.

Symptoms of Internal Bleeding
- Bruised, swollen, or tender abdomen
- Bruises on chest or signs of fractured ribs
- Blood in vomit or bleeding from the rectum
- Abnormal pulse and cool, moist skin

Emergency First-Aid Treatment for Internal Bleeding
- Carefully monitor the patient and be prepared to administer CPR if required.
- Treat the victim for shock, loosen tight clothing and place victim on their side to prevent asperation if they vomit.
- Get the victim to medical assistance.

Open Wounds to the Skin
In this category, anything from a Band-aid to sutures may be necessary. There are five major categories of open wounds:

Abrasions – An abrasion is an injury where the outer surface of skin has been scraped away, such as a scratch or rope burn. There is usually some minor oozing of blood and serum. Depending on how the injury occurred, it is usually contaminated by dirt or foreign matter and in danger of infection.

Incisions – These are the types of wound

caused by any sharp, knife-like object that leaves a clean cut. This category is similar to surgical incisions where the cut edges are smooth and even.

Lacerations – This class of wound is similar to an incision but with jagged edges due to tearing. Suturing is the common medical procedure.

Puncture – As its name implies, a puncture occurs when a foreign object is pushed into the skin. This could be as simple as a splinter that only penetrates the superficial layers of skin or a nail, sharp stick or fishing hook that penetrates deeper. With this type of wound, you usually will not see much external blood (this, however, does not mean that there is no internal bleeding).

Avulsion – An avulsion is a wound where the skin or a body part has been pulled or torn off. It is a severe traumatic injury and medical assistance should be sought as quickly as possible. As with an amputation, any severed tissue should be saved and taken with the injured person to the hospital.

Emergency First-Aid Treatment for Open Wounds

Abrasions

- Clean the wound with soap and water or other disinfecting cleaner. Use hydrogen peroxide with caution since this can cause minor tissue damage. Be sure to use clean water when flushing the wound!
- Blot the wound dry with a clean and dry cloth or preferably sterile gauze.

- Apply pressure over the injured site for a few minutes to reduce bleeding. Remember to use a dry compress since a wet one will hinder blood coagulation.
- Apply first-aid or antibiotic cream to the abrasion to prevent infection.
- Cover the wound with a Band-aid or bandage. For best protection, the bandage should cover an inch beyond the edges of the wound.
- Apply an ice pack over the final bandage to reduce swelling and relieve discomfort.

Incisions

- Clean the incision.
- Apply pressure to stop the bleeding.
- Use tape or a Steri-Strip skin closure to pull the skin together before applying a dressing. "Butterfly" adhesive strips, made by cutting "V"-shaped notches on both sides of the strip, will place less adhesive area on the wound. (Consider shaving the hair from both sides of the wound before pressing the cut skin together. Skin closures will adhere better.)

Lacerations

- Clean the wound.
- Apply pressure to stop the bleeding.
- Pull the edges of the wound together using skin closures.
- Apply a pressure dressing.
- Seek professional medical assistance since sutures will probably be required.

Puncture
- Clean the wound.
- Apply a pressure dressing.
- Apply an ice pack over the final bandage to reduce swelling and relieve discomfort.
- Seek professional medical care.

Avulsions – If, for example, a finger has been severed, a pressure dressing over the stump to stop bleeding and protect the injury is about all you can do until medical facilities are reached.

One important point concerning serious wound dressings – once a dressing is applied, leave it alone and DO NOT take it off to check the wound. If unnecessarily disturbed, you might undo the positive measures already applied and start the bleeding again.

Tetanus
The severity of an apparently non-bleeding wound can be deceiving since, if you are not protected against tetanus (lockjaw), you are at risk of contracting this serious disorder along with other infections (which may require an antibiotic).

Anyone who spends time outdoors should be aware of the danger of contracting a tetanus infection from a deep, soil-contaminated wound (particularly when working around animals or in areas where the soil is contaminated by animal droppings). Keep your tetanus boosters updated and keep a record of when you had your last one.

Suturing

After rendering first aid for a serious cut or incision, a medical professional may choose to close the wound with sutures. Here is a general summary of what is involved in suturing. Hopefully, it will help to remove some of the mystery concerning this common procedure. WARNING: If you are not trained in this technique, leave it up to professionals.

The Suture – This thread-like material is used to hold severed tissue together. It can be absorbable if used internally or non-absorbable for external use. Some materials used in non-absorbable sutures include silk, cotton, nylon, dermal and stainless steel. One of the reasons why so many different materials are used concerns tissue reaction to foreign materials in the body. The body reacts by rejecting any foreign substance causing a tissue reaction. Stainless steel, for example, is popular in surgery because, of all the suture materials, it evokes the least tissue reaction.

Suture size is also important since different materials and weights of thread are matched to the task and tissues involved. Generally speaking, suture material should not be stronger than the tissues it is expected to hold together. Of all the suture materials, silk and nylon are the most widely used. Size is designated as 2-0 or 00, 3-0 or 000, etc. – the smaller the number, the stronger the material. To hold skin together, a size of 000 or 0000 is generally used. Needles can either be straight or curved, with curved being the most commonly used type.

After the skin around a cut has been sutured, edema or swelling usually occurs and proper suture tension is critical for good healing. If the suture is too tight, swelling will probably make it overly tight, putting stress on the wound.

Gunshot Wounds

This is a special category where first-aid measures are primarily used to stabilize the individual. A lot of critical damage is done when a bullet strikes tissue. Getting the victim to an ambulance or helicopter with trained EMTs or paramedics is of paramount importance.

Emergency First-Aid Treatment for Gunshot Wounds

- Use pressure to slow or stop the bleeding.
- Treat the victim for shock.
- Get the victim to professional medical assistance as soon as possible.

WARNING: Gunshot wounds are extremely dangerous injuries and are all too often fatal. The best "treatment" is prevention. If you shoot, *always* be sure of your target before you pull the trigger!

6. SPRAINS, STRAINS & FRACTURES

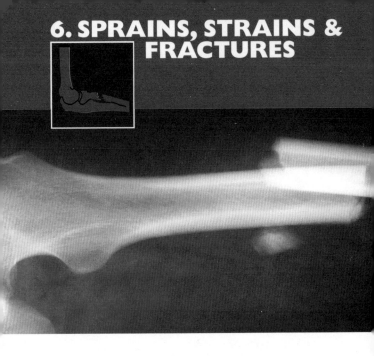

We humans walk upright and gravity insures that we frequently face the possibility of a fall. The result can be something as simple as a pulled muscle or worse, a sprained ankle or broken bone. In any outdoor activity as well, there is always the risk of an unexpected impact injury that can damage bones or connective tissue. While all of these injuries can be equally painful, unless a broken bone is visible or there is distortion of a limb, being able to correctly distinguish between a strain, sprain and fracture could require an x-ray. When such an injury happens, play it safe.

As shown in the x-ray at left, the femur (the "big bone" in the leg), has been fractured and displaced. Securing a broken bone to prevent movement is critical, since rough and sharp edges of a fractured bone can damage tissue and sever blood vessels and nerves.

SPRAINS

A sprain is the result of a ligament or tendon at a joint being stretched or partially torn. A ligament is the piece of fiberous tissue that joins two bones together while tendons are the inelastic fibrous tissue that attach muscle to bone.

Determining whether an injury is a sprain or a fracture is important before applying first-aid.

Symptoms of a Sprain

- Characterized by pain, then tenderness, followed by rapid swelling of the area due to fluid oozing from torn vessels under the skin
- Bruising, skin discoloration or black and blue marks

Emergency First Aid for a Sprain or Fracture

Treatment can be summarized by the letters P.R.I.C.E. Here is what you should do:

- **"P" for PROTECTION** – Use a splint or Ace bandage to immobilize the ankle, being careful not to wrap the area too tightly or cover the toes. If a bandage is too tight, the toes will be constricted and will visibly change color. This means that circulation has been obstructed. A visual inspection is important in determining if all is well. If you cover the toes or fingers you will not be able to see color changes. After a bandage has been applied, additional swelling may occur and even a properly applied bandage may become too tight and must be adjusted.

- **"R" for REST** – Keep your weight off of the injury. If a bone is displaced, the last thing you need is bone fragments damaging other tissue, nerves and blood vessels.
- **"I" for ICE** – Apply ice or a cold pack to the injury for the first 24 to 48 hours. Cold causes blood vessels in the injured area to constrict which lessens oozing of fluids and resultant swelling. Remember, don't apply heat

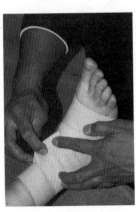

for the first 48 hours! Heat causes the vessels to dilate (vasodilation), which increases the amount of fluid that seeps from broken vessels and swelling will increase.

An ace bandage can help secure a sprained ankle. The elastic bandage will reduce movement and provide pain relief by supporting the ankle.

- **"C" for CHANCE** – There is always a chance that what you believed to be a sprain or a muscle strain is in reality a fracture. If you are not sure, get to your doctor and get an x-ray. Until then, treat all such injuries as potential fractures.
- **"E" for ELEVATION** – Elevate the affected joint or part to reduce swelling by taking pressure off of the injured area. If vessels are ruptured, pressure from fluid adds to the swelling.

MUSCLE STRAINS

This is a common injury in the field. Strains occur as a result of over demand being placed on a muscle or group of muscles. The symptoms are soreness but no loss of strength. Strain becomes more serious when muscle fibers are torn. When this happens, the damage causes the muscles to bleed internally. If the fibers are torn apart, the muscle is considered ruptured.

Emergency First Aid for Muscle Strain
Treatment is similar to that for a sprain or fracture.
- Apply ice for the first 24 hours to reduce swelling.
- Elevate the injured area and wrap it with an Ace bandage to stabilize the injury until the victim can be moved to a medical facility.
- A physician may recommend hot baths after 24–48 hours.

BROKEN BONES & FRACTURES

If you severely injured an area, you may have a broken bone or fracture. Whether the bone is displaced or not, keeping motion to a minimum is critical.

General Types of Fractures
There are two types of fractures, the first of which is the most serious.

Compound or Open – In this case, a piece of broken bone sticks through the skin. Due to this break in the skin, infection is a serious concern, even with good medical care.

Simple or Closed – In this case, the broken bone can be partially or completely broken but is contained within the skin and body tissue. There can, however, be either minimal or severe visible distortion of the injured area as a result of internal dislocation of the bone. Outside contaminants that can cause infection are not usually a concern.

Symptoms of a Fracture
- Intense pain with movement of affected area
- The victim may have difficulty in moving the injured area.
- Bruising
- Swelling
- The injured area looks abnormal when compared to opposite side. The limb is visibly distorted.
- Shock

Emergency First Aid for Fractures

Correct management of this type of injury is critical and any fractured bone must be stabilized. Any wrong movement or further dislocation of the limb or body part can cause severe damage if the fractured area is allowed to move on its own.

- Be careful how you move anyone with a broken bone!
- Follow the P.R.I.C.E. approach as previously stated, (immobilize the injury) and seek medical care as soon as possible.
- A compound fracture must be immobilized but no pressure should be applied to the injured area. Never try to press the protruding bone back into the wound. Any movement or pressure on the protruding bone can cause splintered or sharp bone edges to sever or damage nerves, blood vessels or tissue.
- If there is a potential for spinal injury or fracture, *do not move the victim without support.* There is danger of paralysis if you move a victim of a spinal injury who has not been propely stabilized (immobilized).

What Not to Do

- Don't massage an affected area.
- Don't try to straighten a broken limb.
- Don't allow the patient to move on their own.
- Don't move the joints above and below the fracture.

Splinting

Any suspected fracture should be splinted or immobilized. Splints help to prevent further injury and provide pain relief by immobilizing the injury. All injuries should be splinted before the person is moved to reduce the chance of further injury.

Make splints from materials such as branches, boards or even layers of cardboard. Ideally splints should be applied with elastic bandages but emergency wrapping materials can include bandannas, climbing straps, duct tape and clothing or blanket material torn into strips. Splints should be padded and the wraps should securely hold the splint in place. Take care that the dressings are not wrapped so tight as to block circulation.

Check the pulse and sensation below the splint every hour. Whenever possible the joint both above and below a fractured bone should be splinted to protect the break site.

Arm, Shoulder, Elbow, Wrist, Finger – Use a sling to immobilize injuries to the collarbone, shoulder and upper arm. Wrap the sling with a large bandage encircling the chest.

Forearm and Wrist – Apply a straight splint that secures and aligns both sides of the fracture.

Finger – Use small pieces of wood or cardboard or "buddy-tape" to the adjacent fingers.

Pelvis, Hip, Leg, Knee, Ankle, Foot – A person with a broken pelvis or upper leg should be moved only by trained personnel. These breaks can result in dangerous internal bleeding. If you must apply a splint, it should extend to the lower back and down past the knee of the affected side.

Knee Injuries – Splints should extend to the hip and down to the ankle. Apply splints to the back of the leg and buttock.

Ankle and Foot – These can be wrapped alone. Supports can also be used along the back and sides of the ankle to prevent movement. Keep the foot at a right angle in the splint.

Temporary "Buddy Taping" – A lower-leg injury can often be protected by taping the injured leg to the uninjured leg. An injured finger can be secured to the adjacent finger.

TRAUMA TO THE HEAD

When the bones that protect the brain (skull and its substructures) become cracked, be aware of the possibility of an intercranial hematoma (a blood clot between the brain and skull). With such an injury it may take weeks for symptoms to appear. There is also the danger, with a severe impact injury, of swelling of the brain. With all head injuries, see your M.D. or D.O. as quickly as possible.

Symptoms of a Skull Fracture
- A visible deformity of the skull
- Bloody or clear fluid leaking from the ear or nose, which is likely to be the cerebrospinal fluid that surrounds and protects the brain and spinal cord from injury

- Pupils of the eyes unequally or oddly dilated
- Black and blue discoloration or bruising around the eyes and ears, which can indicate blood leaking from a ruptured blood vessel

Emergency First Aid for Skull Fracture

- Keep the patient resting and quiet, since excitement increases apprehension which, in turn, can increase blood pressure.
- Be ready to perform CPR if the injured person stops breathing!
- Seek emergency medical assistance as soon as possible.

Concussion

A brief unconsciousness following an impact injury to the head or neck caused by significant jarring of the brain. Brief unconsciousness is caused by disruption of the brain's electrical signals. How long a person remains unconscious may indicate the severity of the concussion.

Symptoms of a Concussion

- Brief unconsciousness
- Pupils are dilated (enlarged).
- Drowsiness
- Loss of memory
- Blurred vision and/or vomiting
- Headache
- Persistent confusion

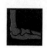

- Convulsions
- Repeated vomiting
- Unusual eye movements
- Muscle weakness on one or both sides

Emergency First Aid for Concussion

- Immediately seek medical care.
- Constantly monitor the individual for the first 24 hours. Even after medical intervention, if you cannot wake the person from sleep, summon help immediately and get that person to the hospital. This may indicate that the person is going into a coma.

Emergency First Aid for Minor Head Injury

- Use ice immediately after the injury to reduce pain and decrease swelling. Bleeding under the scalp, but outside the skull, creates "goose eggs" or large bruises and bumps.
- Apply ice for 20–30 minutes at a time. This can be repeated about every 2–4 hours as needed. Use a light cloth to wrap the ice or apply a commercial ice pack.
- Minor head injuries can be treated in camp as long as someone is available to watch the injured person. Bed rest, fluids and a mild pain reliever such as acetaminophen (Tylenol, etc.) may be given.

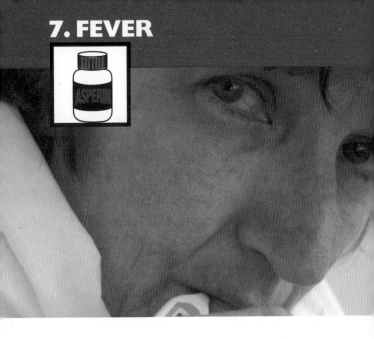

7. FEVER

You feel lousy, and when you take your temperature, you find it elevated. Now the question becomes how high a fever must be to become a major cause for concern. To answer this question, I will provide information on what our body's "normal" temperature should be and what causes changes.

Normal body temperature is arbitrarily defined as 98.6°Fahrenheit or 37°Centigrade. These numbers are only an average. A normal range, which can be influenced by various factors, can be anywhere from 96.8 to even 100°F. Therefore, a significant fever, medically known as Pyrexia, is one where the reading is above 100.4°F or 38.0°C.

Fever is a symptom and not itself an illness. When present, an elevated body temperature can indicate that something is wrong. Elevation of body temperature is one of the body's defense mechanisms against inflammation and infection.

The regulation of body temperature takes place in a part of the brain called the hypothalamus. Depending on the body's need to conserve or eliminate heat, this region of the brain can switch on the temperature regulating mechanisms. These consist of shivering, a reaction that produces heat. Conversly the hypothalamus can command the body to sweat to eliminate heat through evaporation on the skin.

When taking a temperature, there are different choices of thermometers and several places of insertion. One of the most accurate readings is from a rectal or vaginal insertion. A reading of temperature taken by these methods will register a full degree Fahrenheit higher from its normal range when taken by an oral reading. For example, if the mean oral temperature is 98.6°F, then a mean of 99.6°F is what you would expect for a normal rectal reading.

Signs of a Fever
- Sweating and shivering
- Headache and a flushed appearance
- Thirst
- Rapid breathing
- Confusion and delirium, which in extreme cases can lead to seizures

Procedures for Taking a Temperature

- Wash off and "shake down" the thermometer so the mercury reads below 98°F.
- Place the thermometer under the tongue and do not bite down.
- Keep the thermometer constantly in place for 3–5 minutes.
- Use soap and cold water to wash the thermometer before storage.

Causes of Fever

In considering an elevated temperature, we can find a wide range of potential causes. Out in the field, unless the cause is obvious, the origin of a fever can be difficult to determine. Whatever its origin, remember that a fever is an indication that someting is wrong and should always be a cause for concern.

The most common causes of fever have a bacterial or viral basis. When there is a bacterial infection, proper diagnosis and the prescription of an appropriate antibiotic can usually work to eliminate the underlying problem.

Since not all causes for a rise in body temperature are easily diagnosed, you may need to consult a physician. In order to properly make a diagnosis, the doctor will probably need to order a series of tests and apply proper diagnostic and reasoning skills. Therefore, if you are on your own, don't ignore a severe fever and seek assistance.

Emergency First-Aid Treatment for Fever

- Rehydrate – replace lost fluid. Drink a lot of water or fruit juice.
- With a severe fever, sponge the victim down with water (not alcohol) to cool down the body. Apply an ice pack to the forehead.
- Rest and avoid strenuous activity that might further elevate temperature.
- Administer antipyretic medication (aspirin, acetaminophen etc.). Be careful with children under the age of 16 since they are susceptible to a rare disorder called Reye's Syndrome that can cause liver and brain damage. This disorder can be associated with taking aspirin during a viral infection.
- If you have a fever lasting over 2–3 days, you should consult a physician or seek emergency medical assistance.

8. STINGS, SNAKE BITE & POISON

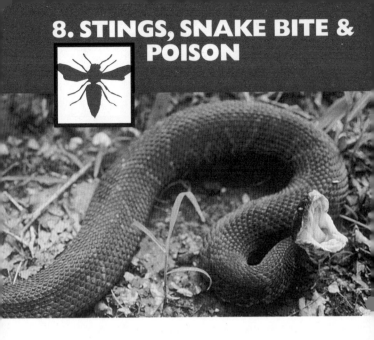

The 16th Edition of *The Merck Manual of Diagnosis and Therapy* states that "while it may take over 100 bees to inflict a lethal dose of venom in most adults, one sting can cause a fatal anaphylactic reaction in a hypersensitive person." In fact, *Merk* goes on to state that there are 3–4 times more deaths in the United States as a result of bee stings than those that result from venomous snake bites.

Despite this, snake bite is a danger that persons in the outdoors can face if they are not careful, especially in warm climates such as in the Southern states. Although statistics concerning snakebites are not exact, it has been stated in the

Merck Manual that over 45,000 individuals every year are bitten by snakes, of which less than 8,000 are from venomous varieties.

The *Merk Manual* goes on to state that "fewer than 15 fatalities per year occur, mostly in children or the elderly, in untreated or under-treated cases." This low fatality rate is attributed to the quick availability of medical care and the fact that a venomous snake does not always fully inject venom when it bites. In the United States, most bites come from the snakes classified as pit vipers. These species include rattlesnakes, copperheads and water moccasins.

ALLERGIC REACTIONS

An anaphylactic (allergic) reaction is a reaction that can happen once a person's immune system has been sensitized – exposed to something foreign to the body. When exposed again, the body mounts a faster and stronger immune reaction and an immune response is possible. This is why even a person who has not been allergic before can experience an allergic reaction weeks or even years later. This can mean unfortunately that no one is safe from an allergic reaction all the time.

During an allergic reaction, histamine causes vasodilation in the victim. Blood pressure and circulating blood volume must be restored to normal to avoid shock.

If you know you are allergic, your doctor may

prescribe a bee sting kit. This usually includes alcohol swabs, a tourniquet, chewable antihistamine tablets and a syringe pre-filled with aqueous epinephrine. The epinephrine has a vasoconstrictor effect which counteracts the histamine being released in the body and restores the pressure and blood volume by constricting the capillary bed. Always read the enclosed information before it is needed and follow your physician's suggestions on how and when to use it.

Be aware that the allergic responses from other venomous bites and stings such as from hornets, fire ants, spiders and other insects can be similar to the stings of bees/wasps. This also applies to the allergic reaction to non-venomous bites from mosquitoes, flies and fleas.

Symptoms of Insect Stings and Bites

Normal

- Localized inflammatory response and some minor swelling and redness around the area of the sting

Abnormal – indicates an anaphylactic reaction

- Hives (urticaria)
- Flushing (paleness) of the skin
- Angioedema, sudden painless swelling apparent on the face, hands, feet, etc. Symptoms may include the feeling of a lump in the throat – an indication of swelling. This can lead to wheezing and can affect breathing.

- Gastrointestinal symptoms – vomiting, nausea, diarrhea and "gut" pain
- Watering of the eyes, sneezing and rhinorrhea (a mucus discharge from the nose)
- Seizures, hypotension (low blood pressure), faintness and vascular collapse

Emergency First Aid for Stings and Bites

- Remove the stinger, if present, by gently scraping the stinger out of the skin. Do not pinch it; this may inject any venom left in the sack.
- Wash the area of the sting with soap and cold water. Keeping something cold on the sting will keep the swelling down and can prevent the venom from spreading.
- Apply an antihistamine like Benadryl or calamine lotion to the area. A topical analgesic may relieve pain and itching.
- Consult with your physician about taking an over-the-counter antihistamine such as Benadryl to relieve some of the symptoms.
- If you know you are allergic, and carry a bee sting kit, use it according to your doctor's direction and the instructions included in the kit.

TICKS

Two diseases associated with tick bites are Lyme disease and Rocky Mountain spotted fever. Lyme disease, commonly contracted in the outdoors, between May and October, is caused by a spirochete (a spiral shaped bacterium), known as *Borrelia burgdorferi* and is carried by a pin-head sized tick, *Ixodes dammini*, also known as the deer tick. Not all ticks carry Lyme disease or *Lyme borreliosis*. Lyme disease has been reported in 47 states, with most cases occuring in the Northeast region of the United States.

The threat of Lyme disease is most likely during the early months of warm weather, May and June, a time when ticks are in their nymph stage and are most likely to transmit the disease. Although June is the peak time of transmission, you are still at risk all through the summer months. If you spend a lot of time in the outdoors, ask your physician about the feasability of receiving the Lyme vaccine.

Rocky Mountain spotted fever is another tick-born disease that occurs in the United States, Mexico and in Central and South America. The disease is caused by a bacteria known as *Rickettsia rickettsii*.

The disease can be difficult to diagnose in the early stages, and without prompt treatment it can be fatal. Because the bacteria infects the cells lining blood vessels throughout the body, this disease may involve the respiratory, central nervous, gastrointestinal, or renal systems.

Precautions
- Use a tick repellent in areas known for ticks.
- Wear light colored clothing, so as to better be able to spot a tick.

- Wear long sleeve shirts and trousers, tuck your pants into your socks or wear tick gators.
- Repellents containing permethrin can be sprayed on boots and clothing. Repellents containing DEET can be applied to the skin. Use DEET with caution on children.
- Perform a frequent body check for ticks.
- Check pets since they may carry the tick and can also become infected.
- Remove ticks with tweezers by grasping them on the mouth end and not over the central gut area. Thoroughly disinfect the bite site and wash your hands with soap and water.

Symptoms of Lyme Disease

First Stage – following the tick bite
- A red rash (erythema chronicum migrans) that may look like a bull's eye may appear at the sight of the bite.
- Flu-like symptoms
- Swollen lymph nodes (regional lymphadenopathy)

Second Stage – appears from weeks to months after a bite
- Severe headache
- Joint and body aches and pains plus swelling, similar to severe arthritis
- Chills & fever
- Fatigue for no apparent reason
- Memory loss, poor concentration and possible dizziness

- Eye & ear pain
- Heart palpitations

Third Stage – occurs weeks to years after bite

- Arthritis
- Neurological problems
- Skin disease

If you believe you may have contracted Lyme disease, contact your physician as soon as possible.

Symptoms of
Rocky Mountain Spotted Fever

- Fever, nausea, vomiting, severe headache, muscle pain, lack of appetite
- A rash first appears 2-5 days after the onset of fever – it begins as small, flat, pink, spots on the wrists, forearms and ankles. These spots eventually become raised on the skin.

Later Symptoms

- Rash, abdominal pain, joint pain, diarrhea
- Red, spotted rash after the sixth day

SNAKE BITE
Precautions

- Be alert to your surroundings.
- Don't put your hands where you cannot see when climbing or reaching into holes.
- Look before stepping over a rock or log.
- If going to an unfamiliar area, inquire ahead of time as to what snakes are common and where to go for emergency medical aid if bitten.
- Wear snake-proof chaps or boots.

Symptoms of Venomous Snake Bite

Snake venom is a complex mixture made up of proteins which can cause the following:

- The bite of a pit viper should show one to six (depending on the number of times struck) single or double fang puncture wounds.
- The area may swell and pain will become quite severe almost immediately.
- Local tissue, blood vessel and cell damage
- Neurological and coagulation defects which can cause bleeding in the lungs, kidneys, peritoneum and heart

Emergency First-Aid Treatment for Venomous Snake Bite

- Keep the snake bite victim at rest.
- Loosely immobilize the injured part in a functional position, just below heart level.
- Remove all rings, watches and tight clothing.
- Get the patient to the hospital as quickly as possible. If the snake is dead, bring it to the hospital so that the physicians can determine the proper antivenin to administer. Be aware, however, that even a dead snake can be dangerous. There can still be venom in the fangs which can be injected by muscle reaction.

Nonpoisonous Snake Bite

- Wash the area with soap and water and call your doctor for advice.

POISON

The accidental ingestion of a poison is unlikely by those who are old enough to read this book. Yet 33 percent of home injuries are due to poisoning. In the following section, I will cover what to look for if you suspect that someone has accidentally ingested poison. Poisons can include over-the-counter and prescription medications and household cleaning materials and chemicals.

A dangerous and deadly form of poisoning that can affect persons involved is carbon monoxide poisoning. Carbon monoxide (CO) is a colorless, odorless, poisonous gas produced by the incomplete burning of various fuels. Appliances fueled with natural gas, oil, kerosene, coal or wood may produce carbon monoxide. Burning charcoal and running cars also produce carbon monoxide.

If you are using a kerosene or other fuel combustion space heater to heat your cabin or tent, or spend time in an RV or other vehicle, you may be at risk. Remember, never use an open flame or portable fuel-burning stove inside a tent and never burn charcoal inside a tent or other enclosed space.

Poison First-Aid Kit Should Contain:
- Activated Charcoal
- Syrup of Ipecac

Signs and Symptoms of Poisoning

- Chemical burns and swelling around the mouth
- Mild to severe forms of nausea, vomiting, diarrhea and abdominal pain
- Confusion, a rapid heart beat
- Seizure and a loss of consciousness

Emergency First-Aid Treatment for Poisoning

- Call the Poison Control Center or hospital emergency room for immediate advice (keep these telephone numbers accessible). Tell the emergency personnel that you have a poison first-aid kit and what it contains.
- Get the victim to a medical facility as soon as possible.
- Examine the mouth for chemical burns and swelling that might hamper breathing.
- Do not offer anything to drink or try to induce vomiting.
- Make sure the victim can breathe.
- Be prepared to give CPR if breathing stops.
- If approved by a physician, use your poison kit to administer a tablespoon of Syrup of Ipecac or a glass of warm water or milk. If vomiting does not occur in 20 minutes, you may be told to repeat this, but only once. Afterwards, give 2 tablespoons of Activated Charcoal in a glass of water and wait for medical assistance.

- Gather evidence of the possible ingested substance to help in providing adequate treatment.

Symptoms of Carbon Monoxide Poisoning

- Flu-like symptoms without the fever
- Headache
- Fatigue
- Shortness of breath
- Nausea
- Dizziness & confusion

Emergency First-Aid Treatment for Carbon Monoxide Poisoning

- Get the victim fresh air immediately.
- Seek medical assistance.

POISON IVY, OAK & SUMAC

Poison ivy, oak and sumac are "poison" plants that cause allergic skin reactions. They grow almost everywhere in the United States, except Alaska, Hawaii and some desert areas. Poison ivy generally grows east of the Rocky Mountains while poison oak grows in the Western and Southeastern states, Canada and Mexico. Poison sumac grows in the Eastern states and southern Canada.

You can identify poison ivy by its compound leaves with three leaflets. Poison oak has three lobe-leafed leaflets that make up each leaf. Poison sumac has a row of seven to 13 paired leaflets and is found in swampy areas in the Northeast and Midwest and Southeast.

The rash is caused by what physicians call allergic contact dermatitis. It is an itchy rash caused by contact with urushiol, an irritating oil contained in the plants' sap. You can get this rash by touching the sap of the plants or touching something that has the sap on it. You can also get a reaction by being in the smoke from burning poison plants.

About 85 percent of all people who come into contact with urushiol develop allergic reactions. Scratching poison ivy blisters will not spread the rash. However, scratching the blisters can lead to a bacterial infection.

Symptoms of Poison Plant Allergy
- Allergic reaction usually appears within 12 to 48 hours
- Severe itching, redness and swelling, followed by blisters
- Blisters become crusted.

Emergency First Aid for Poison Plant Rash
- Wash exposed areas with cold running water as soon as possible.
- Apply an over-the-counter lotion – calamine lotion, Burow's solution (aluminum acetate).
- A lukewarm bath with oatmeal or baking soda may ease itching and dry oozing blisters.

9. HEAT & COLD

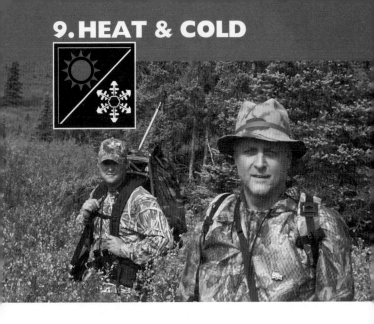

A burn is damage to the skin or other parts of the body caused by contact with flame, extreme heat, hot objects or caustic chemicals. Damage to the skin, present in all categories of burn, can predispose the victim to infection at the surface site of the burn as well as internally.

In addition to the intensity, the area of the burn is important and is usually measured in terms of a percentage of total body area that has been burnt. Burns covering more than 15 percent of the body's total surface area can lead to shock and require immediate medical attention. Physicians use special antiseptic creams for serious burns, including silver nitrate and mafenide acetate preparations.

The author on a caribou hunt in Alaska. Despite the northern latitude, there was as much exposure to ultraviolet radiation as on a beach in Florida. Here, a wide brimmed hat protects the face and ears from sunburn.

BURNS

Burns and their treatment are catagorized by type, area, location, depth and severity. Burn depth is categorized as first, second or third degree. The required first-aid treatment will depend on the category of the burn.

Symptoms of Burn Categories

First Degree

- Skin is red in color, similar to a sunburn.
- Sensation is intact and somewhat painful.
- Minor inflammation and fluid accumulation in and around burn

Second Degree

- Skin is red in color.
- Skin is blistered.
- Pain is more intense.
- Inflammation and fluid accumulation in and around burn

Third Degree

- Skin dark red and charred or may be gray or white in color
- No sensation or pain
- Fluid accumulation and inflammation in and around burn

Emergency First-Aid Treatment for Burns

- Remove constricting items like rings and wristwatches.
- Irrigate (dowse) the burned area with cool water.
- Clean the area gently with chlorhexidine solution.
- Treat first degree burns with local skin care such as aloe vera.
- Apply topical antibiotic.
- Cover burnt area with a sterile dressing or cling film (burn dressing).

For more severe burns (second and third degree)

- Seek immediate evaluation by a medical professional or physician.
- Monitor patient for shock.

NOTE

- Don't apply ice to a burn (can cause additional tissue injury).
- Don't apply creams, lotions to severe burns.
- Don't apply butter or oils to a burn.
- Don't burst skin blisters or remove skin.

DISORDERS ASSOCIATED WITH HEAT

Exposure to Sunlight

Too much of a good thing, specifically over-exposure to ultraviolet B (UVB) rays from the sun, can be dangerous. The ultraviolet (UV) wavelengths that the earth constantly receives from the sun are shorter than those of visible light and, over time, have a damaging effect on living tissue. According to *Primary Care Secrets*, "fair-skinned individuals should be advised to minimize exposure from 11:00 a.m. to 2:30 p.m., times when about 70 percent of harmful ultraviolet radiation occurs." Don't be fooled into thinking that you are safe on a cloudy or foggy day, these conditions aren't good UV filters, and you can still get burned.

Sunburn

When we are overexposed to high levels of ultraviolet B (UVB) rays, areas of the skin can become red, swollen and painful. This is due to congestion in the capillaries (the small vessels that connects arterioles and venules) that supply blood to our skin. This effect can take place from one to 24 hours after exposure. Later, blisters may form and the damaged area of skin may peel.

A person suffering from sunburn may also experience chills, fevers, weakness and lowered blood pressure. In extreme cases, shock is possible.

The real danger, however, is the cumulative effect, which over time, can cause cancers, skin discolorations and a disorder called actinic keratosis, a condition where scaly gray to dark pink and wart-like patches appear on areas where you were heavily exposed to sun.

An increased risk of skin cancers, such as

squamous and basal cell carcinoma and malignant melanoma is a possibility. If you have moles that have changed shape, color and size, get them checked by your doctor. In fact, get any suspicious or new blemish on the skin checked by your physician.

Photosensitivity

There are those who experience an exaggerated sunburn reaction after only a short exposure to the sun. In some cases, this can be the result of taking certain medications. These include specific diuretics, antifungal agents and antibiotics (including the common antibiotic tetracycline). To be safe you need to know the effects of medications you may be taking.

Prevention

Stay out of direct sunlight – easier said than done in the outdoors. Clothing can filter some dangerous rays. Wear a wide brimmed hat and use sunglasses. It is an excellent idea to use sun screen. It should be water-proof and have a sun protection factor (SPF) of at least 15.

Emergency First-Aid Treatment for Sunburn

Mild Sunburn

- Take a cool shower.
- Apply first-aid sunburn cream. These will usually contain hydrocortisone.

- Don't break watery blisters. This opens the area to infection and hinders healing. If they do break, remove the skin fragments and apply a first-aid antibiotic cream.
- Some physicians recommend taking an anti-inflammatory medication as Aspirin to reduce the swelling and discomfort.

Severe Sunburns
- Follow the above suggestions and contact your physician for advanced treatment options.

Stresses of Heat

Usually our bodies can maintain a normal range of temperature by sweating. Sweat evaporates off the surface off the skin, cooling the body. This process helps to regulate internal temperature. When this system fails due to excessive exertion or exposure to heat, there is the possibility of contracting one of the "heat emergency" conditions that are commonly referred to as heatstroke, sunstroke and heat exhaustion.

Our body's primary protection against heat-related disorders is the ability to perspire. If we become dehydrated, consume too much alcohol, take certain medications or are involved in heavy physical exercise, this ability can be severely compromised with drastic results. The resulting failure of the body's heat loss mechanisms can have an abrupt onset and can quickly turn into a very dangerous medical emergency!

Salt loss

Dehydration depletes the system's electrolytes and plasma volume. Overweight and older individuals are at greater risk. It should also be restated that if you are taking certain medications, such as those for motion sickness, edema, asthma or irritable bowel, you may be at a greater risk for heatstroke.

Heatstroke (Sunstroke)

Heatstroke is a major threat. In the United States nearly 4,000 people each summer die as a result of it. In severe cases the victim's body temperature can rise to more than 104°F and can cause widespread cellular injury and multi-system organ failure.

When dealing with heat stroke, emergency help should be summoned as soon as possible since the condition can become deadly within minutes.

Symptoms of Heatstroke

- Skin is hot and dry to the touch and has a red coloration (person appeaers flushed)
- Rapid & shallow respiration
- Rapid heart beat
- Confusion
- Dizziness (vertigo)
- Headache and exhaustion
- Body temperature around 105°F
- Blood pressure either high or low

Emergency First-Aid Treatment for Heatstroke

- Call for emergency medical assistance.
- Get the victim out of the sun.
- Start the cooling down process as soon as possible. Fan the person and use water to cool them down gradually but steadily in order to drop the body temperature to at least 101°F.

Heat Exhaustion

This is also known as heat collapse or heat prostration. As with the sunstroke, excessive sweating due to exertion on humid and hot days can deplete the body's electrolytes and plasma volume. This can lead to heat exhaustion.

Heat exhaustion can begin with excessive sweating. This can lead to dehydration and to circulatory collapse which can turn into a progressively dangerous situation.

Note that sodium chloride (salt) tablets can irritate the stomach and cause edema (swelling) when taken in high doses in certain individuals. CAUTION: If the first-aid treatment does not seem to help, get professional assistance or call your physician for advice.

Symptoms of Heat Exhaustion

- Generalized malaise
- Cold and clammy skin
- Headache

- Nausea & vomiting
- Rapid heartbeat
- Increasing weakness and fatigue

Emergency First-Aid Treatment for Heat Exhaustion

- Get the victim out of the sun or heat and into shade or a cooler area.
- Lie the person down and slightly elevate the feet.
- Give the victim water to drink (not ice water), to help to restore the body's fluid volume. Electrolyte solutions, such as Gatorade, are very effective.
- Give them something salty to eat such as potato chips.

Heat Cramps

These are severe cramps or pain in the muscles that result from excessive sweating brought about by high temperatures and/or physical exertion.

Due to sweating, the body looses sodium and occasionally magnesium and potassium.

Oddly enough, heat cramps are also a possibility among those who participate in winter sports such as skiing. They can occur when someone over-dresses on cold days while participating in a lot of body heat generating physical activity. This is also why hunters need a layered approach for dressing so they will not overheat and perspire.

Symptoms of Heat Cramps
- Profuse perspiration
- "Knotted" feeling and cramps in the muscles, especially in the extremities
- Acute abdominal pain
- Skin is either dry, hot, cool or clammy

Emergency First-Aid Treatment for Sunstroke
- Have the victim rest.
- Massage affected muscles.
- Drink liquids to replace electrolytes.

DISORDERS ASSOCIATED WITH COLD & WIND

Hypothermia

If you hunt big game in the fall nearly anywhere in North America, you should be prepared for temperatures that can range from below 0°F to the 50s and possibly even 70s. Both can be uncomfortable with the former having the real possibility of becoming deadly due to a disorder called hypothermia. Hypothermia means that the body tem-

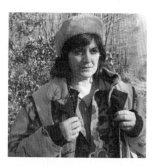

Dressing in layers is an important technique in managing comfort and safety during outdoor activities in cold weather. By removing layers of clothing, you can aviod excessive sweatiing during exertion and add layers to stay warm when stationary.

perature is lower than what it normally should be.

Since hypothermia comes on gradually and can be deadly at "deer hunting" temperatures, between 30 and 50°F, one can become a victim before he knows what is happening. This makes hypothermia a threat for hunters, skiers and anyone who works or plays in the outdoors in cold temperatures. This disorder can set in before you realize what is happening. Hypothermia can be a killer. Danger factors for hypothermia include outdoor temperature, wind speed, being wet and wearing improper clothing.

Hypothermia simply means that the body's temperature falls below what is considered normal. To diagnose this disorder, the temperature of an affected person would be below 95°F. If this happens and the body cannot increase its temperature, the result is death to the cells and tissues due to ice crystals forming in the soft tissue and fluids of the skin.

Symptoms of Hypothermia
- The victim feels cold.
- Uncontrollable shivering
- Tiredness and slurred speech
- Loss of balance
- Disorientation, confusion & hallucinations

Emergency First-Aid Treatment for Hypothermia
- Get the victim into a warm environment. Start a fire and make or provide a shelter.

- Get the person into dry clothing.
- Warm the person.

How to Neutralize Avoidable Causes of Hypothermia

Wear a Hat in Cold Weather – Depending on what text you read, an uncovered head will lose anywhere from 20 to 60 percent of the body's heat. Even if it is only 20 percent, that's a lot! Keep your head, ears and, if possible, your face covered when out in the cold.

Dress in Layers – By wearing layered clothing, when you exert yourself you can simply open your jacket and/or remove a layer of clothing to regulate heat. Layered clothing permits you to adjust protection to suit the situations you encounter.

Stay Dry – If you are dressed too warmly, movement and exertion will cause you to perspire. Within a short period, the clothes nearest your skin become damp. When you cease physical activity in cold weather, damp clothing will cause you to rapidly lose body heat and begin to shiver. You may then be at risk of hypothermia.

To avoid this, plan trips in cold conditions carefully to avoid overexertion. Layered clothing will help manage body temperature and help you avoid becoming soaked with perspiration. In the field, dry your boots nightly since your feet perspire during the day. Damp boots are poor insulators and will accelerate heat loss and you will rapidly experience the effects of lost body heat.

Another danger is getting wet by being caught in a rain storm without proper protection. If you lack rain clothing, carry a large plastic garbage bag with you, since it is lightweight and can provide some protection as a makeshift rain garment.

Get Enough Sleep – When you are tired, your judgment can be impaired and physically, you are more susceptible to the effects of cold weather.

Poor Conditioning – If you are out of shape, just walking in heavy clothing and carrying equipment can be difficult. Exertion when one is out of shape results in excessive sweating and susceptibility to cold.

Nutrition – The body produces heat from the energy it gets from the foods we eat. When outdoors in cold weather, select foods that the body can metabolize more quickly, such as carbohydrates and sugars. I find it beneficial in cold weather to snack all day to keep a steady flow of fuel to help to build up body heat.

Be Aware – When you are alert to potential problems, you are less likely to venture into the cold without being properly prepared. This includes realizing that as we age, the sensitivity to cold is sometimes not as great as it would be to someone younger. This, along with the possibility of not being able to recover from a decreasing body temperature as quickly or easily as a younger person, increases the danger of hypothermia.

Frostbite
This is a common injury caused by extreme cold.

When exposed to extremely low temperatures, the cells of the skin and subcutaneous tissues can freeze. First to be affected are generally the nose, ears, cheeks, fingers, toes or anything that is fully exposed, insufficiently covered or has poor circulation. In extreme cold you must be especially aware of the possibility of frostbite and watch out for signs of tissue injury in yourself and others.

Symptoms of Frostbite
- White and glossy skin caused by blood vessels constricting to save body heat
- Pain can subside and disappear (there is little pain if the tissues are frozen)
- Blisters
- The affected area becomes stiff as a result of the tissues losing their elasticity.
- Tissue necrosis (dead tissue), a result from blood being cut off to the tissue by constricting vessels. This can lead to loss of circulation and gangrene.

Emergency First-Aid Treatment for Frostbite
- Get the victim out of the cold.
- Soak the affected area in warm water, between 98° and 110°F. CAREFUL: If the water is too hot, there is the possibility of causing a burn because the victim's tissue is numb.
- If the individual is conscious, give the affected

person warm, NOT HOT drinks. If they are unconscious, never try to administer liquids by mouth.

- Get the victim to medical help.

What Not to Do

- Don't rub affected hands or other body parts together in an effort to warm them. Friction can damage frozen cells and tissue.
- Don't rub the affected area with snow since it has no purpose! The objective is to warm the tissue, not to keep it cold!
- Don't drink or administer alcohol since alcohol will give a false sense of feeling warmth and can cause loss of muscle coordination. Alcohol is a physical depressant and a vasodilator (expands the blood vessels) which can result in the body losing heat.
- Don't use tobacco since it is a vasoconstrictor (contracts the blood vessels). When the diameter of a vessel is constricted, the smaller diameter hampers circulation. This can raise the blood pressure. Remember, you do not want blood vessels constricted or dilated, but to be of normal size.

Dressing to Prevent Cold Injury

When facing a cold environment, the preparations one makes depends on what you perceive as the potential risks. The "pre-trip adjustments for the perceived conditions" approach is the best plan

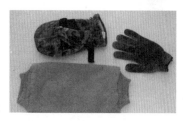

Gloves do not keep your hands as warm as mittens which trap heat from the entire hand. Using a muff with a heat pack will keep your hands warm all day in static outdoor situations.

of action for most situations, as long as you have taken the potential for rapid changes in weather conditions under consideration.

To be comfortable and safe in cold weather when hunting, hiking, or snowmobiling, pay careful attention to your selection of clothing and footwear. Before getting into conditions and appropriate equipment, I will mention a few basics on the selection of equipment and clothing.

To begin with, dark surfaces and dark colored clothing are warmer than light surfaces or light colored materials. To take advantage of environmental heat, stay in bright and non-damp areas out of the wind. Keep track of weather and environmental conditions around you.

Equipment to Stay Warm

Dressing in layers and keeping dry are the obvious factors in staying warm. Remember, if it is cold in one's environment, body cooling is a gradual process when the individual is dry. When wet or damp, body cooling is accelerated. Therefore, you must stay dry. One solution is to pack an inexpensive emergency raincoat with a hood. These

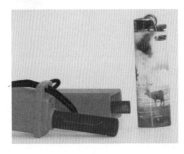

A fire can save your life if you become chilled or lost in the cold. It's a good idea to carry a lighter or a fire starter such as the Strike Force (steel striker) shown at left.

are light, compact and even if it is not raining, can serve as a windbreaker. Put it on under your jacket to trap heat. Unfortunately, they are impermeable and trap perspiration during exercise.

How you dress is important! – Dressing in layers allows you to add or remove items of clothing when appropriate. In cold weather, always wear a hat since anywhere from 20 to 60 percent of the body's heat is lost from the head.

Concerning what material for clothing is best, I try to purchase that with a high percentage of wool since, in my experience, this seems to be the best material to keep warm. Wool is an excellent insulating material and will help to keep you warm even if it's damp.

You can also choose garments made from or lined with one of the modern waterproof synthetic materials like Gore-Tex. Gore-Tex allows body moisture to escape while keeping you dry and warm. In selecting hand coverings, remember that mittens keep you warmer than gloves. If I plan to be sitting a lot, I will put a disposable heat pack into each mitten. This is extremely effective in keeping my hands warm.

Disposable Heating Packs – These easily portable, chemical-reaction, non-toxic heat packs are available from various suppliers. They produce heat for 10 hours on average and come in convenient sizes. Some are cut as boot insoles. The HotHands heating pack gives 130°F to 140°F of warmth and lasts up to 12 hours.

In hypothermia situations, having a heat pack on hand can at least buy time by quickly providing an opportunity to warm up. In an emergency, this could provide enough heat to keep a person from going into full-fledged hypothermia.

NUTRITION

One of the easiest ways to explain the importance of eating to youngsters is to use the example of a wood burning stove. I tell them that for a stove to give off heat, it needs to be fed fuel in the form of wood. They are told to think of their bodies as wood burners and, before venturing out into the cold, to eat a

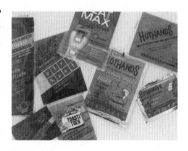

High tech heat packs take up little space and will give off sufficient heat to keep you comfortable. They can also be a valuable first-aid device in preventing and treating hypothermia.

good breakfast as fuel so your body, like the wood burner, can produce heat.

One element for staying warm outdoors involves eating good meals and then snacking in between. When you are trying to build up energy and body heat quickly, eat foods in the carbohydrate category that the body can metabolize quickly.

An active winter hunter or hiker will often burn a minimum of 100 extra food calories per hour, with a light load on flat terrain and up to 500 or more with a heavy load on steep terrain. On a typical winter hunting or hiking trip, you burn up around 2,000 to 3,000 food calories beyond your normal intake. If you are sleeping in a cold tent, you may burn another 1,000 calories just to keep warm at night. Overall, your total daily intake of calories should be 3,500 to 5,000 calories.

Unless you have a complicating physical condition like diabetes, don't worry about gaining weight. While you need to eat a lot of food, you will also burn a lot of calories. While carbohydrates are our best source of quick energy, fats, on the other hand, store up to 200 calories per ounce and provide more long-term energy but take longer to digest. In the backcountry, you will need a sufficient intake of fats to properly use carbohydrates. Proteins provide 80 less calories per ounce, take longer to metabolize and don't metabolize directly into blood sugars.

High-Energy Foods
- Candy – Milky Way, Snickers, Pay Day, Reese's Pieces, M&M's, Hershey bars, hard candy, etc.
- Trail Mix
- Dried Fruit
- Granola and granola-based "power bars"
- Crackers

Protein & Fats
- Nuts and Peanut Butter
- Jerky
- Cheese

ATTITUDE

The easiest thing to do in a bad situation is to simply give up. All too often, when a person realizes the full extent of a desperate situation, their first reaction is to panic. On the other hand, someone who has previously thought out what to do in a crisis should probably have the mind-set needed to survive. To prepare yourself in an emergency situation, you need to first shift your thinking from dwelling on mistakes to getting yourself mentally prepared to decide to live and do your best to formulate a plan for survival. Panic and resignation should not be an option!

10. DENTAL CONCERNS

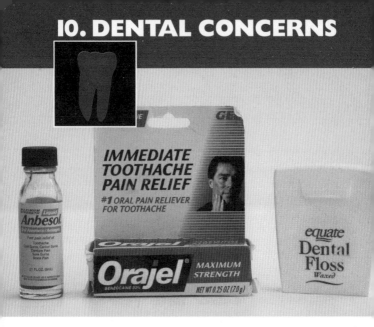

One important aspect of outdoor first aid that many do not consider when putting together a first-aid kit concerns injuries to and problems with our mouth. Here are the disorders, usually caused by some type of mishap, that Dennis P. Marcelli, DDS recommends all should be prepared to handle. What may be frustrating is that the result of certain injuries, as with medical injuries and disorders, can only be corrected in a medical or dental facility where there is high-tech equipment and skilled personnel. Yet, with some of these problems first aid can be helpful.

Most dental injuries or problems that arise in the field will be difficult or impossible to treat without

Various over-the-counter medications are effective in the temporary treatment of broken or painful teeth in the field. A pack of dental floss is a simple remedy for stuck food particles that can cause discomfort.

the proper equipment. This chapter will include simple suggestions to make anyone so affected more comfortable until professional care can be reached.

Falls or blows to the mouth and face can lead to varying degrees of injuries to the teeth, gums, lips, and jaws. These can range from minor scratches and abrasions to severely fractured teeth and jaw.

SOFT TISSUE INJURIES

The soft tissues we are concerned with here are the lips, cheeks, gums and tongue. Injuries to the "outside" skin (cheeks or lips), should be treated in the same way you would treat similar wounds to other parts of the skin. (See Chapter 5)

Mouth & Cheeks

Injuries to tissue on the inside of the mouth and lips will occur in a different type of "skin" called mucosa. Mucosa includes the tissue of the gums, or gingiva, that surround the teeth.

After suffering a wound, be careful how you brush your teeth! Minor wounds inside the mouth, unlike our skin, do not develop scabs. Instead, they are usually covered by a fuzzy, grayish-white layer called a fibrin clot. Removing this clot with vigorous brushing or rinsing will generally delay healing.

Major wounds to internal soft tissues usually require suturing. When the mucosa is cut deeply, it tends to open widely leaving a large gaping wound that often requires sutures. First aid in this case consists of controlling the bleeding with pressure, applying ice or cold compresses to the wound area and then seeking professional help.

First-Aid Treatment for Internal Soft Tissue Injuries

- Rinse the wound gently with clean water or saltwater.
- Apply pressure to the area to stop bleeding.
- Apply cold compresses or an ice pack to the area to reduce or control swelling.
- After such an injury, avoid eating spicy, hard, or acidic foods that might irritate the wound.

The Tongue

This is a large muscle that allows us to speak and swallow and aids us in chewing our food. Damage to the tongue can cause it to swell and create a life threatening airway obstruction. The tongue also has many blood vessels on the underside, and, if injured, it can bleed profusely. Such injuries can commonly happen if you bite your tongue in a fall.

First-Aid Treatment for Wounds to the Tongue – No Bleeding:

- Apply ice chips or cold water to the area.
- Eat a bland, soft diet while it heals.

First-Aid Treatment for Wounds to the Tongue – Bleeding:

- Grasp the tongue between the thumb and forefinger holding a piece of clean cloth or gauze against the wound.
- Apply direct pressure to the wound.
- Apply pressure for 10 to 30 minutes until the bleeding stops.
- Seek medical attention.

Ulcers, Canker Sores & Burns

These are painful and annoying, but not life threatening. They will usually heal without treatment if they are not further irritated. The first step in treating such a condition will be to eliminate any potential irritation if possible.

If the ulcer is caused by a sharp or broken tooth cutting the tongue or cheek, the edge can be gently smoothed with an emery board. Acidic foods, like tomatoes, oranges and vinegar will irritate sores and ulcers and should be avoided. Treatment includes a bland diet, saltwater rinses and milk or butter applied to the areas as a protective coating. Anbesol or related products can be used to relieve pain if available.

HARD TISSUE INJURIES

These "hard tissues" in the mouth are the teeth and jaw bones. The upper teeth are housed in one of the skull bones called the maxilla, and are referred to as maxillary teeth. The lower teeth are anchored in the mandible and are called mandibular teeth. The teeth are anchored to the bone by the periodontal ligament and the bone is covered by gum tissue called gingiva.

Teeth are further divided into groups of anterior (front) teeth, and posterior (back) teeth. The six anterior teeth are comprised of the canines (cuspid or eye teeth), lateral incisors and the central incisors (front teeth). The ten posterior teeth, five per side, starting behind the canines and proceeding to the back of the mouth are the first and second premolars (bicuspids), three molars-first (6 year molar), second (12 year molar) and finally the third molar (wisdom tooth). Thus we have two arches of teeth, the maxillary (upper) and mandibular (lower) with 16 teeth in each arch for a total of 32 permanent teeth.

Children younger than age six have primary or baby teeth. There are ten teeth in each arch, six anterior teeth and two primary molars on each side for a total of 20 primary or baby teeth. Older children and adolescents will have a mixture of primary and permanent teeth.

A tooth is comprised of dentin, which makes up most of the tooth, and the dental pulp or nerve which feeds and keeps the tooth alive. A tooth includes the enamel which covers the dentin where the tooth sticks out of the gum.

Falls or blows to the mouth can lead to varying degrees of injury to the teeth and jaw.

Emergency First-Aid Treatment for Teeth

In the case of a tooth that has been knocked loose, but not displaced or chipped, there is little or no treatment besides avoiding irritating the tender area while it heals. You can apply ice or cold compresses to treat swelling of the lips and gums and take an OTC pain reliever such as Aspirin or Tylenol for pain and soreness. The tooth should be checked and x-rayed upon return from the field.

The next type of injury is a loosened tooth that has been displaced. In this case, the tooth should be repositioned as soon as possible and immediate professional treatment should be sought. With this kind of injury, there will probably be a fracture of the jaw bone that should be evaluated, and the status of the tooth's nerve must also be determined. As a result of an injury of this type, root canal therapy may be necessary.

The most severe injury of this type is a tooth that has been completely knocked out of the mouth (avulsed). In this case, the tooth must be found and any dirt or debris gently rinsed from it. Do not scrub or scrape the tooth, simply rinse away the dirt with clean water. This tooth must be replaced in its socket within 30 minutes, since the chances for successful re-plantation diminish drastically after that. If help can be reached in this time constraint, the tooth can be stored in milk or held under the patients tongue until it can be replanted.

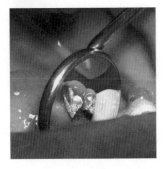

This damaged filling is the result of biting on hard candy, something many of us take with us when hunting or fishing.

If help is too far away, the patient or a companion must replace the tooth. To do this, grasp the tooth with clean hands and push it back into its socket, trying to get it as close to its original position as possible. Once this has been accomplished, have the patient bite down to see if it has been replaced correctly and allows them to properly close their mouth. Repeat this until it is re-positioned the best it can be. The tooth can then be held in place by biting on a clean handkerchief or cloth while going for professional help, which will be needed as soon as possible. The tooth will definitely need to be splinted and stabilized until it reattaches. It will then need root canal therapy and constant monitoring. It is not necessary to replant a primary or baby tooth that has been knocked out for obvious reasons.

Traumatic injuries – This class of wound can present multiple problems. As a result of a fall, an individual may have fallen and hit his mouth on a rock. He has a split and swelling lip, and his front tooth is chipped and pushed backward into his mouth. Treat the bleeding lip first by applying pressure and, if available, cold compresses for the swelling. After that, grasp the displaced tooth with clean hands and gently pull it back into position. The chip will probably need to be ignored for now, unless the nerve is exposed. You will need to get him to an emergency room or dentist immediately with such an injury.

First-Aid Treatments for Minor Tooth Injuries

Injuries to the teeth can include fractures or chips of differing sizes and severity. Small chips that do not involve the nerve may be smoothed by an emery board if they have sharp edges sharp and are cutting the lips or cheeks. Larger fractures that involve the nerve will be very painful and will require dental treatment. One can apply oil of cloves or a topical anesthetic such as Anbesol until professional help is available.

A Lost Filling or Loose Crown – A lost filling can be treated in the field using a temporary over-the-counter filling material until the filling can be properly restored. The cavity can also be filled with cotton or candle wax (not hot wax) as a temporary measure. If there is a sharp edge cutting the lips or cheeks, use an emery board to gently smooth it. Never use metal files or rotary grinders to smooth a sharp edge.

A loose crown or cap can be replaced on the tooth using a temporary filling material, denture adhesive or even petroleum jelly. All of these will hold it in place for a while, but care must be taken not to swallow the loose crown while eating. Never use "super glues" to cement a loose crown or filling, they are toxic and can cause abscesses.

Abscessed Tooth or Gum

An abscess, a pus-filled cavity usually caused by a bacterial infection, is a serious problem and must be treated as such. An oral abscess manifests itself through pain and swelling of the mouth and face, often accompanied by fever, malaise and nausea. Abcesses require professional treatment immediately. An oral abscess can become life threatening in cases where it causes swelling under the tongue and closes the airway. Abscesses of the gum caused by food or foreign bodies caught between the teeth can be treated by gentle flossing to dislodge the object and provide some relief. All of these conditions will require professional dental care, antibiotics and possible extraction or root canal therapy.

Emergency First-Aid for an Abscessed Tooth or Gum

- Apply ice or cold compresses to reduce swelling.
- Apply antibiotics if available.
- Rinse the mouth with warm salt water.
- Administer pain medication (Aspirin, Tylenol or Ibuprofen).
- Seek medical assistance.

Orthodontic Problems

Problems with orthodontic appliances (braces) can arise when you are far from home. Falls and bumps can loosen brackets and wires. A single loose bracket can usually be slid back into place, or it can be removed from the arch wire.

Arch wires are usually attached to the brackets by an elastic or stainless steel ligature. To remove a damaged elastic ligature, place a straight pin under the elastic and pry it from the corners of the bracket. Stainless steel ligatures require cutting the fine wire (fingernail clippers work fine) and unwrapping the wire from the bracket. The loose brackets can then be removed from the mouth.

If the arch wire comes out of the brackets, it can also be cut with fingernail clippers. Cut the wire close to the back of the last bracket to which it is still attached, to prevent the cut end from scratching the lips and cheek. If you have to perform any alterations to the braces, have the brace wearer see their orthodontist immediately upon returning home.

11. PROTECTING YOUR EYES & EARS

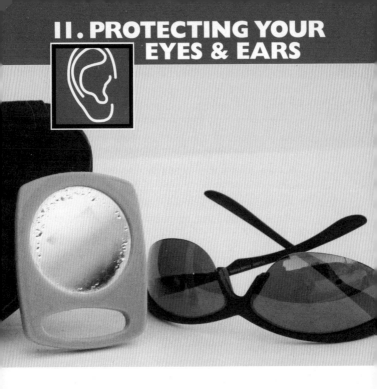

When comparing the senses of sight and hearing, the ability to see is obviously the most important to one's ability to participate in wilderness activities. The capacity to hear is certainly important but not as critical as sight. With "sound proof plugs" in your ears, you can still carry on pretty much as usual. On the other hand, put on blinders for an hour and you will quickly realize that everything will quickly take on a drastically different "perspective" – or lack thereof!

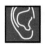

Good safety glasses should be shatter proof and come with additional lenses. A small mirror is handy if you find that you need to remove a foreign object from your eye.

THE EYE, EYE SAFETY AND ASSOCIATED DISORDERS

Many men and women working in factories throughout the United States do not wear protective glasses, even though O.S.H.A. regulations require them to be used in high-risk areas. In addition, there are many operators of small equipment, like chain saws, who feel that goggles are more of a nuisance than they're worth. They, like some shooters, don't take eye protection seriously.

When I use a chain saw, I use a fine wire mesh eye mask attached to my hard hat that does not fog up like goggles. I can see perfectly well through it and my eyes are protected. There is always some kind of eye protection available that makes all of the excuses for not using protection not valid.

Target shooting, chopping wood and splitting logs are just a few of the more obvious activities that can pose dangers to your sight. There are also many non-obvious risks of injury that can affect our ability to see and we should learn what they are and be aware of them. One major serious risk involves injury to the eyes as a result of overexposure to ultraviolet light.

We can get into trouble by not protecting our eyes long before any of the effects of this injury become apparent.

Ultraviolet Protection

The corneal epithelium, the transparent membrane that covers the colored part of the eye, can be damaged and inflamed as a result of prolonged exposure to ultraviolet radiation. Medically, the resulting condition of tearing, photophobia and delayed severe eye pain, is referred to as actinic or ultraviolet keratitis. It is also commonly known as snow blindness. Activities that take place in areas where sunlight reflects off of various surfaces, such as snow and water in skiing or boating, increases the exposure of the eye to sunlight. Repeated episodes can cause sores, permanent scarring and numbness of the cornea.

To treat this condition, you need professional help, ideally from an ophthalmologist. This condition is usually treated as a corneal abrasion.

For first aid, until you can reach medical care, keep the patient's eyes closed and patched. According to *Current*

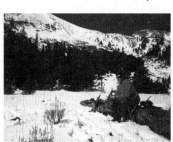

The intensification of ultraviolet light reflected off of snow can cause the condition known as snow blindness. Protective glasses are a necessary safety choice for a wide range of outdoor activities.

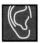

Medical Diagnosis and Treatment, while the condition is painful, the effected individual should recover without complications within about 1 to 2 days.

Long term exposure to ultraviolet radiation radiation (UVR) can also damage the eyes and for this reason, *good* sunglasses should be worn whenever you are at work or play outdoors, especially on sunny days. Be aware that the concept "*good*" is important to your protection. Just because the lenses of a pair of sunglasses are dark does not mean that they offer sufficient protection from these potentially harmful rays.

If you are going to be in the sun a lot, then I would highly recommend that you purchase glasses that offer 100 percent protection from UVR. You will pay more for these but they are worth the additional cost to protect your eyesight.

Impact Resistance – Any hunter, shooter or anyone using power tools, should have sufficient protection that will prevent a fast moving particle from penetrating or shattering the lens. When purchasing eye protection, make sure this important factor is stated by the manufacturer.

What Color Lens is Best? – This depends on your preferences and the conditions where the glasses will be used. What lens is best for what situation? Following are the recommendations according to a chart I obtained from Bushnell, a leading lens manufacturer:

Lens Color	Situation
Yellow	Cloudy and hazy days
Green	Moderate brightness
Gray	Strong, bright sunlight
Clear	Eye protection
Polarized Gray	To reduce glare and metal reflections
Vermillion	Increases contrast for skeet and trap shooters
Photochromic Gray	A good general outdoor lens that gets darker or lighter depending on the available light
Amber	To block all UV and blue light

Symptoms of Ultraviolet Keratitis (Snow Blindness)

- Redness of the eye
- Pain or "gritty" feeling in the eyes
- Inflammation of the eyelid
- Sensitivity to light
- Decrease in vision

Emergency First-Aid Treatment for Ultraviolet Keratitis

- Cover the eyes with thick, moist dressings to cool them and keep light out.
- Secure dressings in place and seek medical help.
- Reassure the victim that the condition will heal in a few days without permanent damage.

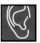

Medical Conditions of the Eyes

The first and most common first-aid problem is a foreign body in the eye. When you are out in the wind, it is not uncommon to have a piece of dirt blown into your eye, or perhaps a small insect might fly in during the evening. Any intrusion is annoying and must be removed.

A speck of grit in the eye gets to be more than an annoyance when the object is hard and sharp and has the potential to scratch the outer surface of the eye. WARNING: When something gets in your eye, do not rub it, rather keep your eye closed or, better still, cover the eye with a dressing to avoid blinking until the object can be removed.

If you are lucky and the speck of matter is under the lower lid, it can be easily seen and removed by gently touching and removing it with a piece of moist gauze or the end of a handkerchief. But first you have to be able to see it. This is why I highly recommend that every hunter or fisherman carry a small mirror in his or her back pack to be used in such an emergency. Remember, there is not always someone around when you need help.

Removing a foreign body from under the upper lid can present you with a little more difficulty. First, try to flush it out with tears by simply pulling the upper lid gently down over the lower lid and holding it there until the tears begin to run. This usually works, but if not, seek medical assistance.

If you are out of reach of a medical facility, you or a friend may have to remove the particle to avoid damage to the eye. This is fine as long as the object is located under the lid and not lodged in the eye. If it is the latter, you must get to an ophthalmologist as soon as possible.

If an object is under the upper eyelid, follow this procedure to locate it, which should allow you or a friend to remove it.

Emergency First-Aid Treatment for a Foreign Body in the Eye

- Have the patient look down.
- Gently grab hold of the eyelash.
- Place a cotton swab in the center of the eyelid and turn the lid up and over the swab.
- If there is a small insect or piece of dirt visible, gently touch it with a piece of moistened and preferably sterile gauze.
- Remove the object when it adheres to the gauze.

Chemical Contamination

Although it is unlikely to occur in the wilderness, if you ever get a dangerous chemical of some sort in your eye, flush it out of the eye immediatly with clean water for 15 to 30 minutes and then get to medical assistance as soon as possible.

Eye Infection

Infections of the eyes, such as blepharitis (infected eyelid), conjunctivitis (pink eye) and a hordeolum

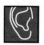

(sty) can be irritating and require medical intervention that will include the application of eye drops or ointment.

Trauma to the Eye

What is generally termed a "black eye" is caused when small blood vessels around the eye are broken, usually when the area has suffered a trauma of some kind, such as being struck by a blunt object. As a result, small amounts of blood leak into the tissues under the skin resulting in a bruise.

The application of cold to the injury, in the form of a cold pack, or even ice, snow wrapped in a clean cloth, should reduce any swelling and discoloration. When you apply ice or a cold pack avoid applying too much pressure to the injured area. You don't want to aggravate the injury.

According to the severity of the blow, however, there may be more damage than you at first realized. This could include a skull fracture (to the fine bones around the eye socket) and potential damage to the optic nerve or even the brain. You may need medical intervention, so when in doubt, get to an emergency room as soon as possible.

In a remote area all that non-medical personnel should handle is the simple removal of foreign bodies from the eye. For lacerations, punctures or other penetrating injuries, gently cover the wound with sterile gauze to prevent eye movement and further injury and immediately get the patient to medical care.

HEARING & HEARING PROTECTION

Did you hear that? Fortunately for most of us, we can reply to that question with a yes. But if we fail to reply, then perhaps we have a hearing problem. If you are becoming hearing impaired, you should get to a physician for an evaluation.

The cause for your hearing difficulty could be a sensorineural hearing loss, also referred to as nerve deafness, a serious condition. It may, however, be caused by conductive (middle ear) hearing loss, the most common cause of which is a blockage caused by a build up of ear wax. This latter type of hearing loss can be easily corrected while the former cannot. Once you find out what the problem is, primarily if it is sensorineural, think back and reflect on the possible causes.

For example, if you do a lot of work with noisy equipment or participate in shooting sports without the benefit of ear protection, these are potential causes that could have been prevented. Unfortunately, at this point, you are taking action after a certain amount of damage has been done.

We frequently take our senses for granted and fail to protect the gifts we were born with. It isn't until one of our senses is compromised that we realize just how precious and important it was. Just ask anyone who lost his or her sight or the ability to hear well and they will usually tell you that they should have been more careful.

Unhappily, preventable injuries will continue as long as man ignores common sense practices and doesn't take safety seriously. As you are probably already aware, there are more ways to abuse these senses than at a gun range. Because of this, what I will be covering here will hopefully make you more aware of the damaging effects of loud noises and indicate what you can do to protect your hearing.

Anatomy of the Ear

The sensory organs critical for hearing and balance, the ears, are anatomically located on the sides of our head. What is visible and referred to as "the ear" is medically designated as the outer ear. This is one of three parts that makes up the total hearing mechanism.

The outer ear is referred to anatomically as the pinna. It consists of a flap of skin and cartridge that acts as a funnel to collect sounds into the external auditory meatus or canal. This canal is about 1 inch long and contained within it are hairs and a lining of wax that functions to trap dirt and foreign objects. This wax also keeps the eardrum moist and flexible.

The second part of the ear is referred to as the middle ear. It is an air-filled chamber behind the eardrum, anatomically referred to as the tympanic membrane. This is the delicate tissue that stretches across the outer entrance of the chamber. We hear when the sound waves reach the eardrum and it vibrates.

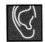

From here, the vibrations continue on to the small bones called ossicles that span the chamber. They are referred to as the hammer, incus and stirrup. From here, with some amplification, the sound vibrations continue on to the cochlea. This is a snail-shaped tube that is the receptor for hearing. Eventually, the sound wave reaches the cochlea nerve and then the brain.

Role of the Ear in Balance

Balance, at least staying upright, requires our muscles to be under control of the brain. To do this, the part of the brain called the cerebellum has the job of taking the information it receives from the eyes (position), sensory nerves in the muscles and joints (also position) and semicircular canals of the labyrinth of the inner ear (detects general movement and head movement). The cerebellum sorts out all of this information and signals the muscles to relax or contract to correct balance. This is why someone with an

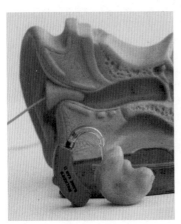

One of the most effective ways to protect your hearing is with an ear plug. The "hearing aid" style device in the foreground is a Walker's Game Ear II, a hearing protection device that combines hearing protection with sound selection technology.

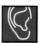

infection of the inner ear, which affects the ability of the inner ear to properly detect motion, may become dizzy or disoriented, a condition called vertigo.

Decibels

Sound is a compression wave traveling through matter. In an airtight chamber, there is nothing to transmit a sound. Therefore, for sound to travel, a medium is necessary and a common one is air. The unit used in comparing sound pressure is the decibel (db). On this scale, 0 is on the bottom and, as the sound progresses, the numbers get higher.

Electronic Ear Protection

Bob Walker, president of Walker's Game Ear, developed a hearing enhancement device that amplifies high frequency sounds. With a high decibel noise such as a gun shot, a safety circuit automatically shuts out all noise levels above 110 db. This means that with properly placed Game Ears, you can hear better and not have to worry about the potentially damaging long-term effect of a firearm blast or other high decibel sounds.

Caliber	Decibel Level
.22 Rifle	145
.357 Magnum	160
.45 ACP	165
.44 Magnum	170

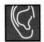

Sound	Decibel Level
Wristwatch near the ear	25
Conversation	65
Vacuum Cleaner	80
Pneumatic chipper	125
50 HP Siren from 100 feet	140

In addition to the Walker Game Ear, various electronic muffs are available. When using electronic hearing devices/muffs in the field, your ears will not ring after a shot and your hearing ability will be enhanced during the hunt.

Standard Sound Muffling Devices

The following gear, while not as elaborate as state-of-the-art electronic devices, will do the job. The objective is to use something that will prevent or reduce sound waves from entering the auditory canal. This can range from a piece of cotton to an ear muff which completely encloses the ear.

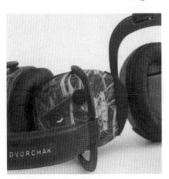

Commercial ear plugs, when properly inserted, have a noise reduction rating of 20 to 30 db and,

Ear muff style hearing protectors, such as these RidgeLine Pro Ears, offer sound management technology and keep your ears warm as well.

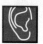

some muffs, up to around 40 dBs. When both are used the effectiveness is increased. However, using one protection device with a rating of 20 and another with 30 does not add up to a protection of 50.

Cotton in the ears is probably one of the simplest and cheapest approaches. Ear plugs are the next best with muffs offering the highest level of protection as long as there is a good seal. Glasses or a lot of hair under the cushions on the muff make the seal less effective, so with muffs alone, you may not be getting the protection you were looking for. In this situation, plugs and muffs help!

What to Look for When Purchasing Equipment

When purchasing ear protection, look for the NRR or noise reduction rating that a particular product offers. The way dB is explained is through the following example. If an environmental noise at the ear is 92 dB and the NRR is 17 dB, then the level of noise entering the ear is approximately equal to 75 dB.

12. HYDRATION

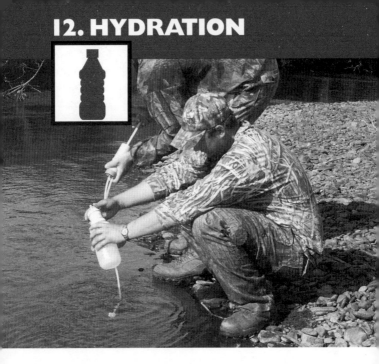

According to the 16th Edition of the *Merck Manual*, an obese adult male's total body water comprises 55 percent of his body weight. The water content in a thin individual is around 65 percent. For women, these values are dropped by 10 percent. Any way you look at it, we are made up of a lot of water which must be constantly replenished for a person to continue to live. The problem is that few of us drink adequate amounts of any liquid at all.

What is "adequate" and why do we need to constantly replenish our body's fluids? To answer

the first part of the question: It is generally recommended that the average individual, meaning a
man who weighs around 150 pounds, should drink
about 96 ounces of water per day. This sounds like
a lot of liquid and it is! Ninety-six ounces is broken
down into twelve full 8-ounce glasses of water.
Then, for every 15 pounds of additional weight, it
is generally recommended to consume an additional 8 ounces up to a maximum of 128. What sex
you are also comes into play when calculating your
intake goal since if you are a 120 pound female, an
intake of 64 ounces per day can be sufficient.

In broad terms, our body needs all of this water
because it uses and excretes large amounts daily in
order to perform functions necessary to sustain life.
The common ways of losing water is through necessary body processes such as exhaling, perspiration and urination. In the simple act of breathing, the
lungs must be moist for oxygen to be successfully
exchanged with carbon dioxide.

This is why you might be more comfortable with a
humidifier when the house air is dry, especially if you
have a breathing problem. Because the body needs
water to help eliminate body wastes, you tend to
become constipated when dehydrated.

It is possible to experience dehydration without
becoming thirsty, particularly if you are involved
in some kind of strenuous activity that is absorb-
ing all of your attention. You will find that you
might be able to get away with not eating much,
even though food intake is important – especially

in cold weather – but you cannot skimp on the intake of fluids that your body requires.

Symptoms of Dehydration

1–5 Percent Deficiency
- Increased pulse rate
- Fatigue, nausea & loss of appetite
- Dark urine or constipation
- Thirst

6–10 Percent Deficiency
- Headache & dizziness
- Difficulty in breathing
- Tingling sensation
- Absence of salivation
- Difficulty walking
- Bluish or grayish skin color

11–20 Percent Deficiency
- Swollen tongue, inability to swallow
- Poor vision
- Shriveled skin
- Delirium, unconsciousness & death

Emergency First-Aid Treatment for Dehydration

Mild cases – Drink liquids & keep warm.

Severe cases – Seek professional medical aid.

Liquids

In choosing the liquid that is preferred for hydration, there is nothing better than water, water and more water. Water is the best liquid to consume when hunting, hiking or simply replenishing the fluids your body has lost through the processes of sweat and respiration. It is generally recommended that you should avoid drinks that contain a high percentage of sugar and artificial chemicals. With drinks high in sugar, you need to drink even more water in order to both metabolize the sugar and satisfy your thirst.

There are other drinks that, if possible, should be avoided or at least their intake reduced. These are beverages containing caffeine, such as tea or coffee. Hunting camps are notorious for making very potent coffee and I advise that your intake should be limited to one cup or less per day. Caffeine is a diuretic, which increases urination by interfering with the normal action of your kidneys by reducing the amount of water and sodium taken back into your blood. With an increase in the rate of urination even more fluid will be lost.

Don't stop caffeinated beverages completely, however, since someone who is used to a few cups a day and abruptly discontinues that practice is liable to experience withdrawal symptoms. The most common of these are mild headaches. Therefore, if you intend to cut out all caffeinated beverages, do so a few weeks before.

High-Altitude Sickness
A lack of fluid is also a factor in what is referred to as high-altitude sickness. This may manifest with signs such as fatigue, headache, tachycardia, dys-

pnea, sleep disturbances and nausea at altitudes as low as 6,500 feet, common elk and mule deer elevations. According to the *Merck Manual*, these symptoms subside within a few days as long as hyperventilation (a means of losing bodily fluid) is not excessive and dehydration is not severe.

Another fact to remember is that hypoxia stimulates breathing. As you ascend to higher elevations, the amount of oxygen in the air is less so your breathing increases to compensate. Due to this physiologic process, more body fluid is lost, fluid that must be replaced if you are to avoid adding stresses to your body from dehydration.

For headaches and exhaustion on high country excursions, take aspirin and stay hydrated by constantly drinking water. Also, get enough sleep and do not overexert yourself for the first few days since it takes a few days to become acclimatized.

Safe Drinking & Washing Water

Don't draw your drinking water from lakes, streams or springs, no matter how clear and clean they appear. Disease-causing microorganisms thrive in waters even in remote areas. Bring your own water supply and replenish it from tested public sources whenever possible. All water of uncertain quality should be treated before using it for drinking, food preparation, washing or brushing teeth. Any water used in a first-aid situation should be as sterile as possible and should be treated to eliminate dangerous organisms.

Boiling

- This is the safest method of treating water.
- Strain water to remove foreign material.
- Heat water to a rolling boil for at least one minute to kill most organisms. Water boiled at high altitude should be boiled longer since water boils at a lower temperature the higher you go.

Chlorination – Bleach

- This treatment will not kill all parasitic organisms. Use regular liquid bleach containing 5.25 to 6.0 percent sodium hypochlorite. Don't use bleach with scents or cleaners.
- Add 16 drops (1/8 teaspoon) of bleach to one gallon of water; let stand for 30 minutes.
- Water should have a slight bleach odor, if it does not, repeat the dosage and let stand an additional 15 minutes.

Purification Tablets & Filters

- Iodine, halazone and other chemical treatment products that do not contain 5.25 percent sodium hypochlorite as the active ingredient are not recommended.
- Follow the directions that come with the tablets.
- Some parasites and larger bacteria are not killed by chemicals and you must also use a water filter. Water filtering devices must be 1 micron absolute or smaller.

13. BOOTS & FOOT CARE

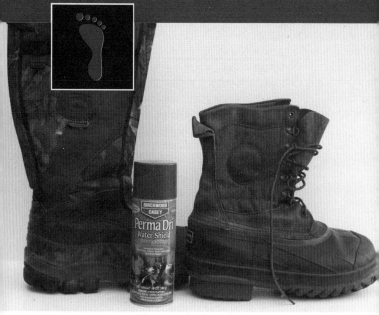

For many of us who hunt, hike or do a lot of walking in the outdoors, some of the most overlooked pieces of equipment center around our feet. At the same time, there are others who are quite serious about hiking and acquire quality equipment by purchasing the right socks, hiking or hunting boots and who appropriately take care of them.

In a state like Pennsylvania, where over a million hunting licenses are sold each year, that single outdoor activity translates into over a million individuals trekking around out there in

Keeping boots in shape is quite important. To take care of mine, I first spray the leather parts with Perma Dri Water Shield, an odorless repellant, which protects leather and fabrics from water and dirt. To the rubber bottoms, I apply a conditioner such as Turtle Wax. This protects the rubber from drying and cracking. I do this twice a year and after each use.

all kinds of weather. It is obvious that some of those million individuals will end up with sore feet after that first day outdoors. Due to sore or blistered feet, there is not a second day or if there is, it is a painful one. Unfortunately many people purchase the right footwear but still end-up with blisters. To avoid these pitfalls, precautions must be taken.

To get advice on this, I asked two individuals in the footwear industry for some of their ideas on foot care and safety. For hunting boots, I spoke with Krystal Krage from Irish Setter Inc. Here are some of her ideas on outdoor boots. Hunting boots can be divided into different categories based on terrain and weather conditions that you expect to encounter. The upper materials, linings, soles and construction are the variables that make these boots perform properly in different environments.

The two primary types of hunting boots are upland boots and big game boots. To properly select a boot, consider what conditions and terrain you'll be walking through, the wetness of the environment, the temperature and the general conditions underfoot.

BOOTS IN GENERAL

The upper is the part of the boot that's above the sole. It supports your ankle and protects your foot. Upper materials are usually leather, or leather combined with tough nylon fabric. Leather provides excellent support and protection and will be sturdier than most fabrics in rocky conditions. Fabric panels, on the other hand, can make the boot more lightweight and flexible. Leather quality can vary quite a bit as well. The top of the line is full-grain waterproof or water resistant leather. Lower-priced boots often incorporate more nylon or use split leathers.

The gusset is the part of the boot where the tongue meets the rest of the boot. This area may be padded for extra comfort when you pull the laces tight to get a secure fit. When you look for a boot, choose one that fits snugly and comfortably so there's less movement of your foot in the boot. Movement within the boot is what leads to "hot spots" or blisters that can make the day seem very long. Pay particular attention to how the widest part of the foot fits in the widest part of the boot and make sure you have the proper width so that toes are not cramped. If you are high-arched or flat-footed, look for boots with addable insoles that allow for more of a custom fit.

Boot Height
Boots come in various heights that offer differ-

ent levels of support. These can range form 7-inch hiker styles to 18-inch snake boots. When selecting a pair of boots, pay attention to where the top of the collar meets your leg. You want a boot that will minimize rubbing! Also feel the padding on the collar and select what feels the best to you. Try on a few different pairs before making a purchase to see which style fits your foot and leg best.

Waterproofing

Waterproofing is extremely important. If you're in the back country with cold, wet feet, it can lead to a medical emergency. If you will be walking through dewy grass in the morning, you may only need water-resistant leather without a waterproofing system. Gore-Tex material is a well known waterproof and breathable waterproofing system used in much outdoor equipment.

Insulation

Insulation is a major consideration in footwear selection. If you're planning to hunt in a warm climate, you'll probably want non-insulated footwear. For cold weather, an insulated boot is desirable. Many boot manufacturers use Thinsulate or Thermolite insulation which is measured in grams. For example, two hundred grams is the least amount of insulation you can buy. Insulation numbers increase from there to 1600 grams. When purchasing a hunting boot, choose your insulation need by the air temperature, ground temperature and the amount of foot movement you anticipate. You'll need to balance your need for a non-sweaty walk with your need for a comfortably warm foot when you're stationary.

Soles

These provide varying levels of traction, cushioning, shock absorption, lateral stability and flexibility. They can be incredibly lightweight and not very durable but you wouldn't want to walk very far in such a boot. Most hiking, backpacking and hunting boots use soles that are somewhere in between. Tread size is also critical when selecting a boot. A shallow tread works best for varying upland terrain where you want to limit the amount of mud and debris that the treads pick up. An aggressive tread with an air bob design works best for mountainous and hilly terrain.

Snakeproofing

Since hunters, fishermen and hikers get into areas

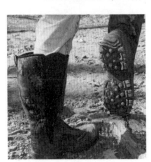

where there are venomous snakes, leg protection is a concern. What makes a boot snake-proof? The best protection comes from

A boot's tread is important and needs to be matched to the terrain. When in slippery mud, you need a tread that will bite in and not slip and performs as a winter tire would in the snow.

tightly woven 1,000 denier basket weave nylon uppers and a snake guard backer. A thorn guard backer is lined through the entire boot for added durability and simply put, the snake guard backer is just a beefed-up version of the thorn guard. From reports by those who have been struck by poisonous snakes, these boots have

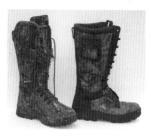

To prevent a potentially deadly bite, when in snake country, wear snake proof boots that, due to their construction, prevent the fangs from puncturing your flesh.

been field tested and they prevented individuals from being bitten. A person struck by a snake while wearing these boots might be a bit shaken, but will not have his skin penetrated by the fangs and will walk away unharmed. If you are going to be in such areas, such protection is simply common sense insurance.

Cordura versus Leather

Another factor to consider when choosing boots is the material from which they are made. Cordura nylon boots have been a hit with hunters and hikers across the country since this material is light-weight and requires little maintenance. Once a Cordura boot gets muddy, simply wash it down with a soft brush and water and when dry, apply a silicon spray to help retain the boots water repellence. On the other hand, when it comes to all leather boots, although heavier, they provide a bit more support and rigidity when in extremely rugged terrain. Also, caring for a leather boot takes a bit more time and treating leather with a conditioner will extend the life of the boot. Then after treating, apply a silicon spray which will help the leather repel water. Basically, no matter what you elect to purchase, you must care for the boot as suggested by the manufacturer and when needed, apply a conditioner and water repellent to assure that your footwear will serve you for many years.

Common Footwear Myths

"If I buy good hunting boots, I don't have to break them in." Not true! The best boots need breaking in. Boots need to conform to your feet, and your feet have to get used to the boots. The sturdiest boots require the longest breaking in, but end up being the most comfortable. Here's another great tip for your feet: get them in shape before the hunting season, not during the hunting season. Get started by walking and constantly increase the distance until you are not out of breadth and your feet feel good in the boot you will be using for hunting. This will put both your feet and body in shape before the season begins.

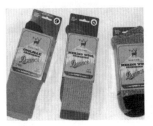

"If your feet are cold, add more socks." The truth of the matter is, the number

Wool or wool blend socks whisk moisture away from the skin while cotton, on the other hand, retains sweat, making your feet feel damp and cold.

of socks you wear has little to do with overall foot warmth. As a matter of fact, the more socks you jam into your boots, the colder your feet will be. Your feet need room to breathe and the better they breathe, the warmer they'll be. The tighter your boots, the faster your feet will get cold since circulation will also be hampered.

Some Rules to Consider About Boots & Socks

- Buy new boots with the socks you plan to wear outdoors to get a proper fit.
- Always wear proper socks.
- Wear a thin liner (polypropylene or Thermax) next to your feet to wick moisture away.
- Next, wear a wool sock! Wool's hollow-core fiber will further wick moisture away from your feet which keeps them dry and warm.

Socks & Boots as Medical Concerns

Before putting on your boots, consider socks. Be careful with designs that have heavy gummed tops meant to hold up your socks. When this is too tight, circulation can be cut when moving, especially in cold weather. You need good blood circulation and don't want to be hampered by the tops of tight socks that turn into a light tourniquet.

Special Concerns for Diabetics – A good pair of shoes or boots can be a healthy choice for everyone but can be a "must" for a few. A major medical concern for those who have diabetes mellitus is the feet, since these individuals are at special risk for foot problems. With diabetes there can be a deterioration of blood vessels and nerves in the hands and feet. This can then limit blood flow to these areas which may lead to gangrene.

If you are a diabetic, be aware of complications to your feet which can manifest as circulatory problems, diabetic neuropathy (along with a decrease in circulation, one may also experience a loss of sensitivity and nerve loss in the feet which due to numbing, affects one's ability to experience pain which can be a warning that something like a blister is forming) and foot infections.

Proper foot care along with proper socks and boot fit is critical for these individuals. It is a good idea for anyone, but especially for diabetics, to examine their feet for any friction rubs and make sure their socks are not bunched and that their footwear fits properly, allowing for unobstructed circulation.

Blisters – These are collections of clear fluid that accumulate in a specific area under the skin. The result is a raised section of skin that is now quite tender and sore. A blister is caused by constant rubbing

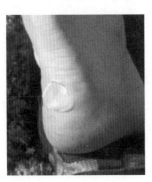

Damp feet and socks and the rubbing of a rough spot in your socks or boot can cause a blister. The ruptured blister above has been dressed with a protective piece of Molefoam to reduce further chafing.

of an area from a shoe that does not properly fit. Large blisters, more than a half-inch in diameter, are medically referred to as bullae. A smaller raised area or blister is referred to as a vesicle. The resulting damage under these rubs are "abused" small blood vessels within the traumatized area. Now what happens is the leaking of serum from these traumatized blood vessels, and the formation of a blister.

The serum is usually sterile and therefore, if the skin of the blister is not broken, the blister provides protection to the area that was damaged by the friction.

By knowing that friction is the enemy that causes a blister, it should be a little easier to prevent them through sensible countermeasures. What first happens in this chain of events is that, as you are walking, friction on an area causes a "hot spot" or "thermal burn." When this happens it soon becomes uncomfortable — this is your body putting out a warning for you to take action or pay later. Again, by understanding that friction is the cause, it becomes evident that further rubbing of that area must be halted. To do this, take off your shoe and sock and cover the area in question with something like smooth surface tape or mole skin.

Remember that the skin on your feet is smooth when dry but becomes tender when hot and wet from perspiration. It is a good idea to carry a second pair of socks so that, if the first pair becomes wet or damp, you can change into a dry pair.

When you put your sock back on, make sure there are no creases in it since this will act like a foreign body in your shoe. Also, inspect and empty out your boot to make sure that there are no irritating objects, such as a pebble or splinter.

If you develop a blister and have to keep walking, a controlled break may be your best bet to reduce discomfort and lessen the chance of more tissue damage if it breaks on its own. Once blisters form, the serum under the skin adds pressure which is quite uncomfortable. You can open and drain the blister using a sterile needle (sterilize the needle by holding it in an open flame), and then cover it with a sterile dressing for a day or two.

Unfortunately, with this treatment you have caused another potential problem. Because the blister was a closed area and the serum was likely sterile, it has now been opened and drained and bacteria can get in through the drainage hole.

Emergency First Aid for a Blister
• Apply a smooth dressing and adjust socks to prevent further irritation.

If You Need to Drain a Blister
• Wash the blistered area with soap and clean water and wipe it with an alcohol swab.
• Drain the blister by making a small opening at the edge using a sterile needle or knife tip.
• Keep the blistered area clean and covered with a sterile dressing.

Moleskin Blister Cushion

For another approach to blister first aid, you can build a cushion with layers of moleskin in which holes have been cut to accommodate the intact blister. If you are worried about infection, or are a diabetic, this may be the best approach. To play it safe, always contact your family physician or podiatrist when you can for their recommendations. Especially if you are a diabetic, you need to contact your health care provider who knows your situation and therefore can best adjust the treatment to your particular circumstances.

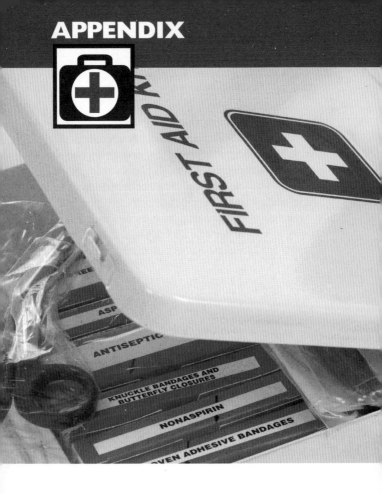

First-aid kits are available in models ranging from basic to very elaborate. Here, you get what you pay for but remember, too much stuff means additional equipment that adds weight and bulk to your gear. You need to make a determination as to what kind of emergencies you might face in the course of the outdoor activities you are planning and assemble your kit accordingly. If you plan to be backpacking, for example, you want a kit that provides the basics but is easy to pack and lightweight to carry. On the other hand, if you are traveling in a vehicle or have a base camp, you might choose a more advanced first-aid kit. Also consider how far you will be from emergency medical assistance and whether or not you have the knowledge and skills to use various types of medical gear.

To find out what is available, go to your local pharmacy or outdoor supplier and look at pre-packaged kits and browse the shelves noting the different categories of first-aid supplies available. Make a list of topics such as basic first aid, foot care, medications, etc. and then go back and purchase what you think you may need or simply would like to have in your kit.

A good way to approach a first-aid kit is to try to keep it compact and light. If you choose to assemble your own kit, there are a wide variety of containers available. These range from backpacks and zipper cases to hard cases and large "tacklebox" style containers. Whatever style of case you choose, it should be waterproof, or at least water resistant.

Again, in deciding what to include in your first-aid kit, make a determination as to what kind of emergency medical situiations you might face and assemble your kit accordingly.

OUTDOORS FIRST-AID KIT

- ❏ Sterile adhesive bandages (Band-Aids) in assorted sizes
- ❏ Latex gloves (2 pairs)
- ❏ 2-inch (2 x 2) sterile gauze pads (4-6)
- ❏ 4-inch (4 x 4) sterile gauze pads (4-6)
- ❏ Triangular bandages (3)
- ❏ 2-inch sterile roller bandages (3 rolls)
- ❏ 3-inch sterile roller bandages (3 rolls)
- ❏ Steri-Strips
- ❏ Hypoallergenic adhesive tape
- ❏ Scissors
- ❏ Tweezers
- ❏ Needle
- ❏ Antiseptic and alcohol wipes
- ❏ Antibiotic spray or ointment
- ❏ Hydrogen peroxide
- ❏ Thermometer
- ❏ Assorted sizes of safety pins
- ❏ Tube of petroleum jelly or other lubricant
- ❏ Waterless hand sanitizer
- ❏ Sunscreen
- ❏ Sanitizing hand wipes
- ❏ Ace bandage
- ❏ Molefoam for blisters
- ❏ Styptic pencil to stop bleeding
- ❏ Tincture of Benzoin in a small bottle with cotton swabs (This enhances the adhesive power of a Steri-Strip or tape to hold a wound together.)

- ❑ Dental floss
- ❑ Large safety pins and a small roll of duct tape
- ❑ Tongue depressors
- ❑ Sling to hold a bandage in place or immobilize a fracture
- ❑ Tick removal kit (magnifying glass and small tweezers)
- ❑ Water purification tablets
- ❑ Small magnifying glass
- ❑ Disposable razor to shave around a wound
- ❑ Heavy-duty fingernail clipper
- ❑ Pencil and note paper
- ❑ Permanent marking pen

Nonprescription Drugs

- ❑ Aspirin or non-aspirin pain reliever such as Tylenol or Ibuphrophin
- ❑ Antidiarrheal medication
- ❑ Antacid such as Pepto-Bismol
- ❑ Laxative and stool softener
- ❑ Allergy medicines
- ❑ Antihistamine such as Benadryl for allergic reactions to poison ivy or insect stings
- ❑ Nasal decongestant – Afrin nasal spray or Vicks Vapor inhaler
- ❑ Cold or flu medications
- ❑ Dramamine (motion sickness)
- ❑ Chap stick
- ❑ Eye drops – Visine or other preparation

- ❏ Toothache medication
- ❏ Paste to fill a broken or painful tooth cavity
- ❏ Calamine lotion for poison ivy & poison oak
- ❏ Antifungal spray
- ❏ Syrup of ipecac (Use if advised by the poison control center.)
- ❏ Activated charcoal (Use if advised by the poison control center.)
- ❏ Aloe vera for minor burns

Prescription Medications

Carry needed prescribed medicines and your schedule for taking them. Carry any pills, in their container and keep them dry. CAUTION – If you have an enlarged prostate, antihistamines can hurt you so consult with your physician about what to use. If you know you are allergic to bee stings, ask your physician to prescribe a bee sting kit (EpiPen).

Other Worthwhile Equipment

- ❏ Flashlight and extra batteries
- ❏ Nonelectric can opener
- ❏ Toilet paper, premoistened wipes
- ❏ Soap, liquid detergent
- ❏ Maps and compass
- ❏ Rain gear
- ❏ Special "survival" or "space" blanket
- ❏ Waterproof matches or fire lighter
- ❏ Pocketknife
- ❏ Plastic trash bags
- ❏ Small shovel and ax or hatchet

PLANNING FOR SURVIVAL

Your most important survival skill is your ability to admit that you are lost or stranded. Once you admit this, get control of yourself, avoid panic and stay calm. Sit down and think. Mentally, you must accept the challenge and make the best of the situation. In most cases, people will be looking for you when it is discovered that you are overdue. To manage panic – STOP – This is the acronym for:

Sit
Think
Observe
Plan

Sit – Sitting down will help keep you from getting into deeper trouble. This can also jump-start the thinking process, and it helps suppress the urge to run or make hasty, foolish decisions.

Think – Survival is the challenge to stay alive and your brain is your best survival tool. In order to survive, you must keep in control by drawing on past training, maintain a positive attitude and develop the will to survive.

Survival Priorities – The Rules of Three:

- You may be doomed in three seconds if you panic.
- You cannot live more than three minutes without oxygen.
- You cannot live more than three hours in temperature extremes without shelter.

- You cannot live more than three days without water.
- You will need food in three weeks.

These priorities tell you that you need to think of the real and immediate dangers, not those conjured up by your fears.

Observe – Observe your surroundings to discover what problems must be solved and what resources you have to solve them. You will need shelter, signals, fire, water and a campsite that is easily spotted.

Plan – Make plans and set them in motion.
- Choose a campsite near an open area or your stalled vehicle.
- Establish a set of signals, with backups, and keep them ready for instant use.
- Construct shelter.
- Gather firewood and start a fire.
- Dispel fears and maintain a positive survival spirit.